Place 2⅛ × 2⅛ **Sticky Notes** here
For a convenient and refillable pad

✓ **HIPAA compliant**
✓ **OSHA compliant**

Waterproof and Reusable
Wipe-Free Pages

Write directly onto any page of *Physical Assessment Check-Off Notes* with a ballpoint pen. Wipe old entries off with an alcohol pad and reuse.

BASICS	MENTAL STATUS	INTEG-UMENT	HEENT	CHEST/BREASTS	CARDIO	ABDOMEN	MUSCULO-SKELETAL
NEURO	UNEXP-FINDS						

Reviewers

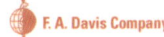
F. A. Davis Company

Always at your side...

Physical Assessment Check-Off Notes

Waterproof and Reusable

Nurse's Clinical Pocket Guide

Brenda Walters Holloway

Includes...

✔ Step-by-step guidelines for physical exams

✔ Only the essential assessment information!

✔ Clinical Documentation tools

✔ Illustrations to enhance assessment techniques

✔ Normal vs. abnormal assessment findings

Contacts • Phone/E-Mail

Name

Ph: e-mail:

Name

Ph: e-mail:

Name

Ph: e-mail:

Name

Ph: e-mail:

Name

Ph: e-mail:

Name

Ph: e-mail:

Name

Ph: e-mail:

Name

Ph: e-mail:

Name

Ph: e-mail:

Physical Assessment Check-Off Notes

Nurse's Clinical Pocket Guide

Brenda Walters Holloway, FNP-BC, DNSc

Purchase additional copies of this book at your health science bookstore or directly from F.A. Davis by shopping online at www.fadavis.com or by calling 800-323-3555 (US) or 800-665-1148 (CAN)

A Davis's Notes Book

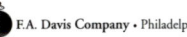

F.A. Davis Company • Philadelphia

F. A. Davis Company
1915 Arch Street
Philadelphia, PA 19103
www.fadavis.com

Printed in China by Imago

Last digit indicates print number: 10 9 8 7 6 5 4 3 2 1

Publisher, Nursing: Robert G. Martone
Developmental Editor: Will Welsh
Director of Content Development: Darlene D. Pedersen
Project Editor: Elizabeth Hart
Design and Illustration Manager: Carolyn O'Brien

As new scientific information becomes available through basic and clinical research, recommended treatments and drug therapies undergo changes. The author(s) and publisher have done everything possible to make this book accurate, up to date, and in accord with accepted standards at the time of publication. The author(s), editors, and publisher are not responsible for errors or omissions or for consequences from application of the book, and make no warranty, expressed or implied, in regard to the contents of the book. Any practice described in this book should be applied by the reader in accordance with professional standards of care used in regard to the unique circumstances that may apply in each situation. The reader is advised always to check product information (package inserts) for changes and new information regarding dose and contraindications before administering any drug. Caution is especially urged when using new or infrequently ordered drugs.

Elizabeth Holman, MSN, RN
Nursing Instructor
RN-BSN Coordinator—Gulf Coast
The University of Southern
Mississippi
Long Beach, Mississippi

Linda Johnson, RN, MSN, DH A©
Assistant Director and Lead
Instructor of the LVN program
Los Medanos College
Pittsburg, California

Paula Kihn, MSN, RN
Assistant Professor of Nursing
Central Wyoming College
Riverton, Wyoming

Rebecca Loth Luetke, BA, BSN,
MSN, RN
Associate Professor of Nursing
Colorado Mountain College
Glenwood Springs, Colorado

Rachel M. Merkel, DNP, RN
Assistant Professor
University of Wisconsin–Eau
Claire
Marshfield, Wisconsin

Connie S. Miller, RNC, MSN
Clinical Assistant Professor
University of Arizona College of
Nursing
Tucson, Arizona

Cynthia L. Moore, MSN, RN,
PLNC
Nursing Faculty
Minnesota State Community and
Technical College
Detroit Lakes, Minnesota

Catharine Muskus, MS, FNP-BC
Assistant Clinical Professor
University of Vermont Dept. of
Nursing
Burlington, Vermont

Grace Nteff, DNP, MS, FNP-BC, RN
Assistant Professor of Nursing
Clayton State University
Morrow, Georgia

Debra Servello, MSN, ACNP
Assistant Professor of Nursing
Rhode Island College
Providence, Rhode Island

Jennifer Sipe, MSN, RN, ANP-BC
Assistant Professor of Nursing
La Salle University
Philadelphia, Pennsylvania

Julie Sterk, RN
Practical Nursing Instructor
Alexandria Technical College
Alexandria, Minnesota

Caitlin Stover, RN, PHCNS-BC
Nursing Instructor
Worcester State College
Worcester, Massachusetts

Margaret Sorrell Trueman, EdD,
MSN, RN, CNE
Assistant Professor
University of North Carolina at
Pembroke
Pembroke, North Carolina

Lizette Villanueva, BSN, M Ed, RN
Lead Faculty
Anamarc Educational Institute
El Paso, Texas

Barbara Wilder, DSN, CRNP
Professor
Auburn University School of
Nursing
Auburn, Alabama

Debra J. Wilson, MSN, FNP, CNL
Associate Professor
CSU Bakersfield
Bakersfield, California

Look for other
Davis's Notes titles!

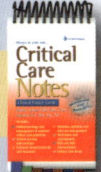

Critical Care Notes
Clinical Pocket Guide

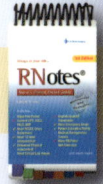

RNotes®
Nurse's Clinical Pocket Guide

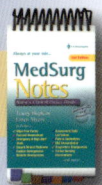

MedSurg Notes
Nurse's Clinical Pocket Guide

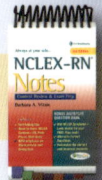

NCLEX-RN® Notes
Content Review & Exam Prep

For a complete list of Davis's Notes
and other titles for health care providers,
visit **www.FADavis.com**.

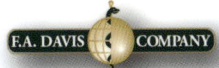

Purpose of This Publication

- A course in health assessment is commonly a required part of preparation for entry into a health-care profession. The "physical assessment check-off exam" is often an essential part of the course.
- The purpose of this book is to guide the student through the specific steps of physical assessment techniques that may be used in the "well-patient physical assessment check-off exam" or in development of the patient's data base.

Features of This Publication

- Numerous photographs and illustrations are included to guide the student through steps of the assessment.
- Examples of an appropriate report for validating expected or "normal" findings are included for each assessment technique.
- Benign variations that may not be common but that do not necessarily represent pathology are cited.
- A section citing unexpected findings and a listing of possible related pathologies has been included in the last tab.
- An overall checklist of assessment steps has been included.
  - The checklist follows the order of the tasks as they are presented in this publication.
  - The program's or class's determined number of points for grading items in the check-off exam may added to a blank column in the list.
  - Blank spaces are left on several rows so that additional skills may be added by the faculty or student.
  - Skills that may not be required for a particular check-off exam may be marked through with an erasable marker.

General Guidelines for Physical Assessment

Order of Assessment

- There is no one "right sequence" in which to perform a physical assessment; attention to patient's comfort should influence the manner and order in which it is conducted.
- Head-to-toe and general-to-specific are used in this guide to physical assessment.
- Skills commonly used in physical assessment are inspection, palpation or touch, percussion (as tapping a drum), and auscultation.
- Inspection precedes performance of other assessment techniques.
- In all areas except abdominal assessment, auscultation is the last skilled used in each area of the assessment.

General Preparation of the Patient

1. Ask patient to empty his or her bladder.
2. Wash your hands.
3. Provide a warm, private environment.
4. Assemble all equipment that will be needed; ensure that all equipment is clean.
5. It is usually appropriate to measure and record patient's height, weight, and vital signs, including blood pressure, before beginning head-to-toe assessment.
6. Provide privacy.
7. Ask patient to disrobe from the waist up and to remove long pants and socks or stockings after you leave the room. Provide appropriate drape(s) to avoid unnecessary exposure.
8. Briefly explain to patient what you will be doing before beginning the physical assessment and as you move through various parts of the assessment.
9. Ensure patient is as comfortable as possible during the entire assessment.
10. Ask patient to let you know if he/she experiences pain or discomfort during the exam.
11. Thank the patient for his/her cooperation when the assessment is completed.

General Equipment Needed

- Felt-tipped marking pen
- Gloves (non-sterile)
- Otoscope and ophthalmoscope attachments for light source (handle)
- Otoscope tips (disposable preferred)
- Pen light (Otoscope light may be used for this purpose)
- Percussion hammer (optional)
- Rosenbaum's pocket eye chart or newspaper
- Scented products with commonly recognized odor for assessment of sense of smell
- Small ruler or tape measure
- Stethoscope
- Tuning fork
- Salt or sugar, substance with bitter taste, and substance with sour taste

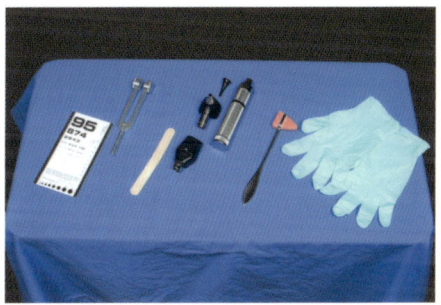

Equipment.

Assessing Mental Status

Prepare Patient
- Patient is seated during the mental status assessment.

Examiner
- Examiner is seated and facing the patient during the mental status assessment.
- Note that if the patient appears withdrawn, wary, or uncomfortable with the examiner, it may be less threatening to the patient for the examiner to sit a little farther away from and at less than a 180° angle to the patient.
- Name 3 colors and tell the patient you will ask him to repeat them in a few minutes. Take note of the 3 colors you asked the patient to remember because you'll be asking the patient to recall them during the memory assessment.

Assessing Level of Consciousness

- Assessed by noting patient's general response to his environment.

Expected Report
- Awake and alert
- Responds appropriately to environment

Unexpected Findings: See p. 162.

Assessing Appearance, Posture, and Grooming

- Note general appearance.
- Note posture.
- Note dress and grooming.

Expected Report
- Neat and clean
- Posture erect
- Dressed appropriately for season and occasion

Unexpected Findings: See p. 162.

Assessing Orientation to Time, Person, and Place

- Ask patient to state:
  - Date
  - Year
  - Name
  - Current location

Expected Report
- Oriented to time, person, and place

Benign Variations
- Patients who have been institutionalized may not know the exact date.
- Patients who were unconscious when admitted may not be aware of their location when initially questioned.

Unexpected Findings: See p. 162.

Assessing Mood/Affect/Behavior

- Observe body for signs of tense muscle tone or quick, jerky responses to sounds.
- Note facial expression.
- Note level of cooperation with health assessment, including eye contact when speaking.

Expected Report
- Appears relaxed, smiles appropriately, and is cooperative with health assessment

Benign Variations
- Patients from some cultures may hold head lowered and avoid eye contact.

Unexpected Findings: See p. 162.

MENTAL STATUS

Assessing Concentration/Attention Span

- Note appropriateness of response to surroundings.
- Note speech pattern for evidence of continuity of thought.

Expected Report
- Attentive to environment; speech demonstrates continuity of ideas

Unexpected Findings: See p. 162.

Assessing Memory

- Name 3 objects and ask patient to repeat them (indicates immediate memory).
- Ask patient to repeat the name of the 3 colors cited when mental status assessment was begun (indicates short-term memory).
- Ask patient the name of the previous president (indicates long term memory).

Expected Report
- Patient displays intact immediate memory by correctly repeating the names of 3 objects.
- Patient displays intact short-term memory by repeating the names of objects cited earlier.
- Patient displays intact long-term memory by stating the name of the previous president.

Unexpected Findings: See p. 162.

Assessing Abstract Thinking

- Ask patient the meaning of a familiar proverb or metaphor, such as:
    - "Don't count your chickens until your eggs hatch."
    - "The grass is always greener on the other side of the fence."

Expected Report
- Patient displays intact abstract reasoning by responding appropriately to common metaphors.

Benign Variations

■ People of different cultures or nationalities may not clearly understand the meaning of all metaphors familiar to the examiner, so if the patient cannot explain the meaning of one abstract statement, try another.

Unexpected Findings: See pp. 162–163.

Assessing Analogies

■ Ask the patient to compare like features of two items. For instance:
   ■ "What is similar about a fork and a spoon?"
   ■ "A puppy is to a dog as a kitten is to a what?"

Expected Report

■ Patient responds appropriately to request to explain analogies.

Unexpected Findings: See p. 163.

Assessing Judgment

■ Ask patient what he or she would do if he were in a burning building or some other hypothetical situation.

Expected Report

■ Patient displays intact judgment by responding appropriately to hypothetical situations.

Unexpected Findings: See p. 163.

Assessing Calculation

■ Ask the patient to count to 56 by 7s or count to 30 by 3s:
   ■ 7, 14, 21, 28, 35, 42, 49, 56
     or
   ■ 3, 6, 9, 12, 15, 18, 21, 24, 27, 30

Expected Report

■ Patient displays intact calculation ability by being able to count to 56 by serial 7s or 30 by serial 3s.

Unexpected Findings: See p. 163.

MENTAL
STATUS

Mental Status Check-Off List

Assessment Task	Performed and Reported Correctly	Performed or Reported Incorrectly	Not Performed
Level of consciousness			
General appearance			
Posture			
Dress and grooming			
Orientation to time			
Orientation to person			
Orientation to place			
Mood			
Affect			
Behavior and cooperation			
Attention to environment			
Concentration, attention span			
Memory: immediate			
Memory: short term			
Memory: long term or remote			
Abstract thinking			
Analogies			
Judgment			
Calculation			

Preparing for the Integumentary Assessment

Gather Equipment
- Light
- Small ruler with mm and cm markings

Prepare Patient
- Explain the procedure.
- The patient is seated and draped with his arms at his side.

Examiner
- Stand in front of the patient, moving to his sides and back to view skin on all body parts.

Assessing the Skin

Inspection
- Inspect skin for:
  - General color
  - Integrity (intactness)
  - Odor
  - Lesions
    - A lesion is any abnormal skin change.
    - Lesions are best visualized with tangential lighting. Tangential means that light is shined "across" the skin.
  - Scars

Palpation
- Palpate (touch) skin to assess:
  - Temperature: Assess with the backs of your fingers.
  - Moisture: Assess with your finger pads.
  - Texture: Assess with your finger pads.
  - Turgor: Assess by pinching a fold of skin over the sternum or inner forearm.
- Note that lesions that are intact and elevated (papular) may be palpated with your gloved fingertips to determine consistency of lesion contents.

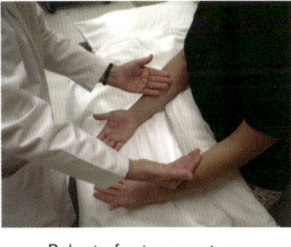

Palpate for temperature.

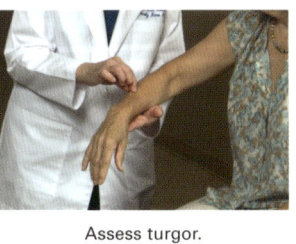

Assess turgor.

Expected Report

- Skin is intact over all body areas and light tan in color with no visible lesions or scars.
- There is no detectable odor.
- Skin is warm, smooth, and moist to touch.
- Skin recoil is immediate with turgor assessment over inner forearm.

Benign Variations

- Skin is black, tan, or pink depending on racial heritage and sun exposure.
- Palms of hands and soles of feet of dark-skinned people may be a lighter color than general skin tone.
- Decreased skin turgor is an expected finding in the elderly.
- Light brown oval macular (birthmark type) lesions with even borders (fewer than 5 in number).
- Scattered nevi (moles) without signs of pathology (see ABCDEs of moles in Unexpected findings section) may be seen over the body and extremities.

Unexpected Findings: See p. 163.

Assessing the Hair and Scalp

Inspection
- Inspect scalp for:
  - Dryness or excess oil
  - Lesions
  - Scars
  - Parasites
- Inspect hair for:
  - Hygiene
  - Color
  - Distribution: If hair is long, lift sections to examine distribution of hair roots.

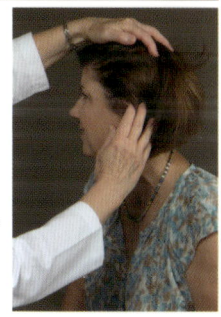

Inspect scalp.

Palpation
- Palpate hair for:
  - Texture
  - Integrity: Roll sections of hair between your fingers and inspect for excessive breakage or fraying of individual hairs.

Expected Report
- Hair and scalp are clean without dryness or excessive oiliness.
- Hair is light brown (or other) in color, evenly distributed over the head, and fine in texture without excessive breakage or fraying.
- No lesions or parasites noted.

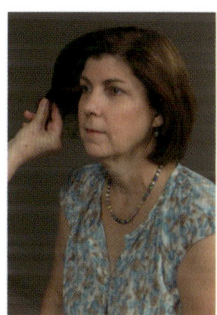

Palpate hair.

Benign Variations
- Hair may vary in color and texture.
- Male or female pattern baldness is symmetrical and is determined by heredity.

Unexpected Findings: See p. 165.

INTEG-UMENT

Assessing the Nails

Inspection and Palpation: Fingernails

- Inspect and palpate fingernails for:
  - Shape
  - Hygiene
  - Nail surfaces (smoothness)
  - Thickness
  - Attachment to nail bed
  - Angle of attachment

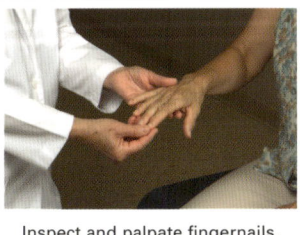

Inspect and palpate fingernails.

Expected Report

- Fingernail edges are rounded and clean with smooth surfaces.
- Fingernails are slightly convex, thin, and transparent with white tips.
- There is no fingernail clubbing, and nails are securely attached to the nail bed.
- Nail-bed angle of attachment measures 160°.

Benign Variations

- Longitudinal ridging of nails is hereditary.
- Nails may be slightly yellowish in color.

Unexpected Findings: See p. 165.

Inspection: Toenails

- Inspect toenails for:
  - Color
  - Nail-bed color
  - Thickness

Expected Report

- Toenails are thin and transparent.
- Toenail bed is pink.

Benign Variations

- Toenails may be slightly yellowish in color.

Unexpected Findings: See p. 165.

Integumentary Assessment Check-Off List

Assessment Task	Performed and Reported Correctly	Performed or Reported Incorrectly	Not Performed
Skin			
Skin color			
Skin integrity			
Skin odor			
Skin lesions			
Skin scars			
Skin temperature			
Skin moisture			
Skin texture			
Skin turgor			
Scalp and Hair			
Scalp, dryness or excess oil			
Scalp lesions			
Scalp, scars			
Scalp, parasites			
Hair, hygiene			
Hair, color			
Hair, distribution			
Hair, texture			
Hair, integrity			
Nails			
Fingernail, shape			
Fingernail, hygiene			
Fingernail, thickness			
Fingernail, color			
Fingernail, angle of attachment			

Continued

INTEG-UMENT

Integumentary Assessment Check-Off List—cont'd

Assessment Task	Performed and Reported Correctly	Performed or Reported Incorrectly	Not Performed
Fingernail, attachment to nail bed			
Toenail: inspection			
Toenail, color			
Toenail bed color			
Toenail, thickness			

Preparing for the Head, Eyes, Ears, Nose & Throat (HEENT) & Neck Assessment

Gather Equipment
- Gloves (determine whether the patient has a latex allergy before choosing gloves)
- Otoscope
- Ophthalmoscope
- Penlight (optional; may use otoscope light)
- Small ruler with cm markings
- Tuning fork
- Two scented items for testing sense of smell
- Items for testing sense of taste: salt or sugar, bitter tasting substance and sour tasting substance

Prepare Patient
- Patient should be seated upright
- Explain procedure

Examiner
- Stand in front of or to the side of the patient.
- Note that cranial nerves (CNs) are usually not tested in chronological order; rather, they are assessed as related parts of the head and neck are assessed.
- Some CNs innervate motor functions, meaning that they control movement.
- Other CNs innervate sensory (senses) functions such as sight, hearing, and detection of touch.
- Some CNs innervate both motor and sensory functions, and different assessment techniques must be used to evaluate the two different CN functions.
- Some nerves have more than one sensory or motor innervation function and, therefore, more than one technique may be needed to assess each separate innervation.

Assessing the Head

Inspection and Palpation
- Inspect and palpate head for:
  - Size
  - Shape
  - Symmetry
  - Lumps
  - Bumps
  - Tenderness
  - Lesions
  - Scars
  - Scaling
  - Parasitic infestation

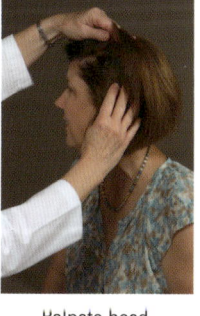

Palpate head.

Expected Report
- Head is symmetrical and appears normocephalic with an oval shape
- Scalp is smooth, nontender, without lumps, bumps, tenderness, lesions, scars, or scaling
- No parasitic infestation is noted

Benign Variations
- Head may be slightly asymmetrical and rounded in shape.

Unexpected Findings: See p. 166.

Assessing the Face

Inspection
- Inspect facial:
  - Symmetry
  - Expression

Expected Report
- Face symmetrical, expression calm

Benign Variations
- Facial features may be slightly asymmetrical.
- Expression may appear anxious in response to the clinical setting.

Unexpected Findings: See p. 166.

CN V: Trigeminal

CN V Motor Function
- Ask patient to clench his teeth together as you palpate the temporomandibular joint (TMJ)
- Evaluate TMJ for:
  - Strength of bite
  - Symmetry of movement

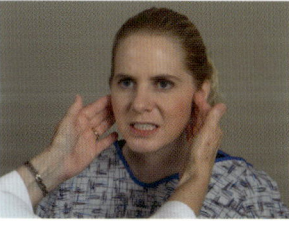
Palpate TMJ.

CN V Sensory Function
- Ask patient to close his eyes, and identify the area touched as you lightly and randomly touch various spots on each side of patient's forehead and cheeks.
  - *Do not establish a predictable pattern while touching different parts of the face.*
- Assess the corneal or the blink reflex by lightly touching the cornea of one eye with a wisp of rolled cotton or by touching the upper lateral eyelash with a gloved finger and while watching for the patient to blink with both eyes.
  - Note that the perception of touch on the cornea or lash is a test of CN V sensory but the actual blink response to touch is a test of CN VII motor.

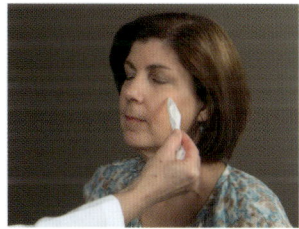
Identify facial areas touched.

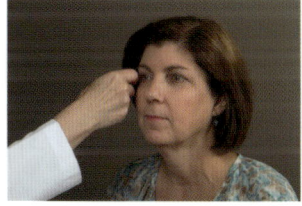
Touch lash to elicit blink reflex.

Expected Report

- Temporal and masseter muscles contract firmly and symmetrically when teeth are clenched.
- Identifies areas touched on each side of face and forehead
- Responds to touch of upper eyelashes by blinking both eyes
- Cranial nerve (CN) V, Trigeminal, motor and sensory intact

Unexpected Findings: See p. 166.

CN VII, Facial

CN VII Motor Function

- Ask patient to:
  - Smile
  - Show teeth
  - Frown
  - Puff cheeks
  - Purse lips
  - Raise eyebrows—note symmetry of eyebrow movement
  - Close eyes tightly

CN VII Sensory Function

- Ask patient to identify taste after placing salt or sugar on anterior aspect of tongue.

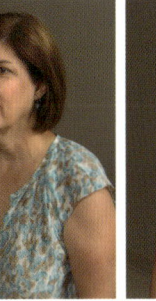
Smile.

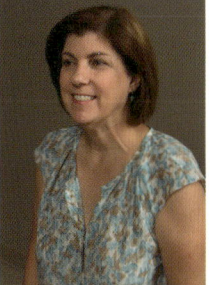
Show teeth.

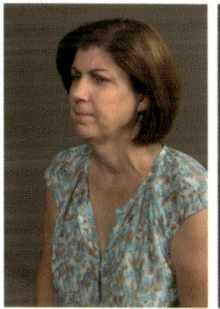

Frown.

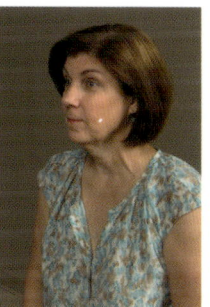

Puff cheeks.

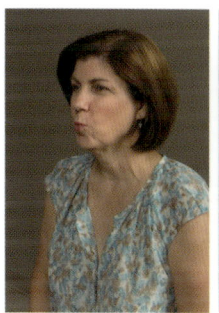

Purse lips.

Raise eyebrows.

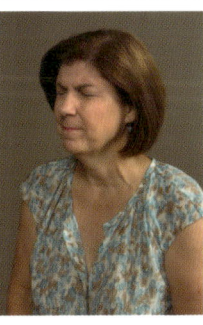

Close eyes tightly.

Expected Report
- Facial muscles move symmetrically as patient makes faces
- Identifies taste of salt or sugar
- CN VII, Facial, motor and sensory intact

Benign Variations
- Facial movements may be slightly asymmetrical

Unexpected Findings: See p. 166.

Assessment of the Eyes

Assessing the Eyebrows, Lashes

Inspection
- Inspect brows for:
  - Quantity
  - Placement
  - Color
- Inspect lashes for:
  - Direction of distal tips

Expected Report

- Moderately dense eyebrows arched along bony prominences above eye orbit; color consistent with hair color
- Lashes turn outward on upper and lower lids
- There is no entropion or ectropion

Benign Variations

- Eyebrows may retain their original color after hair color becomes gray or white.

Unexpected Findings: See p. 166.

Assessing the Eyelids and Lacrimal Apparatus

Inspection

- Inspect eyelids for:
  - Position relative to the eye
  - Lesions
- Inspect lacrimal apparatus for:
  - Swelling
  - Redness
  - Tenderness

Palpation

- Gently palpate each lacrimal apparatus with gloved finger to assess for tenderness.

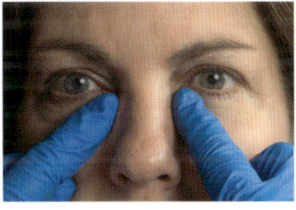

Palpate medial lacrimal apparatus.

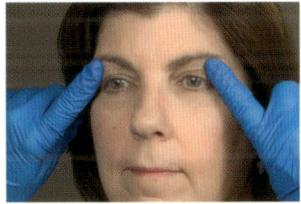

Palpate lateral lacrimal apparatus.

Expected Report
- Eyelids flush against globe of eye
- Lids cover sclera when eyes are closed; upper lids cover 3 mm of irises
- No lesions noted
- No swelling, tenderness, or redness of lacrimal apparatus
- No excess or purulent drainage

Unexpected Findings: See p. 167.

Assessing the Globe of Eye

Inspection
- Inspect globe (eyeball) of eye for protrusion (exophthalmos)

Expected Report
- No protrusion of eye globe

Unexpected Findings: See p. 167.

Assessing the Conjunctiva

Inspection
- Wear gloves when touching tissue around the eyes.
- Gently pull the lower palpebral conjunctiva downward to inspect bulbar (eyeball) and palpebral (inner lid) conjunctiva for:
  - Color
  - Moisture
    - Do not inspect the upper conjunctiva unless patient reports a problem such as pain or a foreign body.

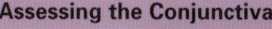

Inspect conjunctiva.

Expected Report
- Bulbar and palpebral conjunctiva pink and moist

Unexpected Findings: See p. 167.

Assessing the Sclera, Iris, Cornea, and Lens

Inspection
- Inspect sclera (white of eye) color.
- Inspect irises (colored part of eye that surrounds the pupil) for:
  - Color
  - Shape
- Assess cornea (tissue that covers the iris and pupil) for transparency.
  - To assess cornea, stand beside patient, and shine light across (use tangential lighting) the globe of the eye.

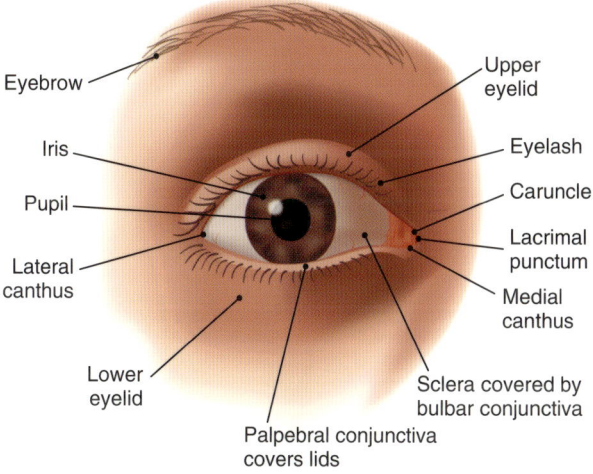

Frontal view of eye and eyelid (Dillon, P. (2007). *Nursing health assessment: A critical thinking case studies approach* (2 ed.). Philadelphia: F. A. Davis Company.

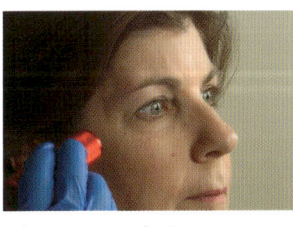

Assess cornea for transparency.

Expected Report
- Sclera white, irises round and blue
- Cornea transparent

Benign Variations
- Sclera may have a slightly yellow or "muddy" appearance in dark-skinned people.
- Irises may be any of a variety of colors and are usually dark in dark-skinned people.

Unexpected Findings: See p. 167.

Assessing the Corneal Light Reflex

Inspection
- Assess the corneal light reflex (also known as Hirschberg corneal reflex) in the following manner:
  1. With a light directed toward patient's nose, ask him to look at a fixed object (not the light).
  2. Assess for equal placement of the light reflection on each eye; the reflection is the corneal light reflex.

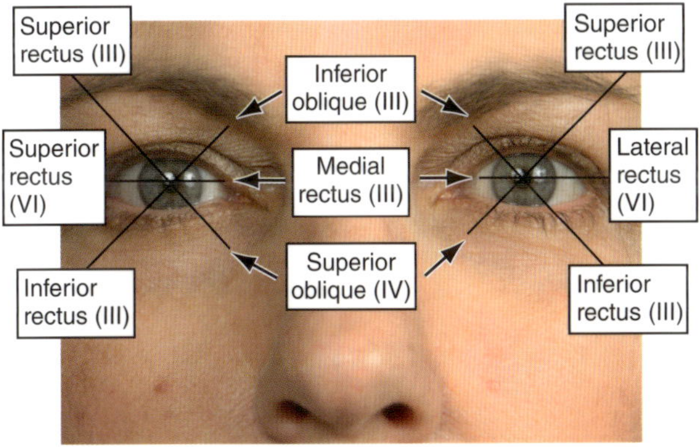

Superior rectus (III)

Superior rectus (III)

Inferior oblique (III)

Superior rectus (VI)

Lateral rectus (VI)

Medial rectus (III)

Inferior rectus (III)

Superior oblique (IV)

Inferior rectus (III)

Corneal light reflex.

Expected Report (Corneal Light Reflex Test)

- Corneal light reflex is symmetrical
- If the corneal light reflection (reflex) is asymmetrical, conduct the **cover-uncover test** in the following manner:
  1. Ask the patient to stare ahead at a fixed object.
  2. Cover one eye, and watch for movement of the uncovered eye to assess whether the eye moves to focus on the object.
  3. Repeat the test on the other eye.
  4. Second, cover one eye, then quickly uncover the eye, and watch for movement of the eye that was just uncovered.
  5. Repeat the test on the other eye.

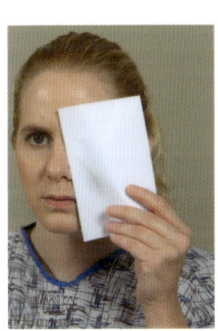

Cover-uncover test.

Expected Report (Cover-Uncover Test)

- Cover-uncover test is negative.

Unexpected Findings: See p. 168.

Unexpected Findings: See p. 168.

HEENT

CN III, Oculomotor

- CN III has three separate motor functions:
  1. Innervates pupillary reaction to light
  2. Innervates 4 of the 6 extraocular muscles (EOMs), which are muscles involved with eye movement
  3. Innervates eyelid muscle

Inspection

- Estimate size of pupils
  - Shining the light on the eye from the side and slowly moving the light to the front of the eye makes pupils easier to see in a person with dark irises.

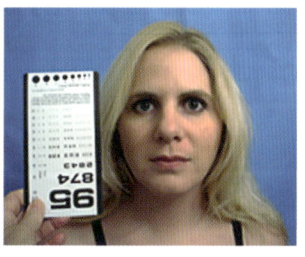

Estimate pupil size.

- Assess pupillary light reflex to:
  - **Direct light:** Shine a light on the left pupil, and watch for it to constrict. Repeat the test on the right pupil.
  - **Indirect light:** Shine a light on the left pupil, and watch for the contralateral (right) pupil to constrict. Repeat the test by shining the light on the right pupil and watching the left pupil for constriction. Pupillary constriction in response to indirect light is known as a *consensual response*.

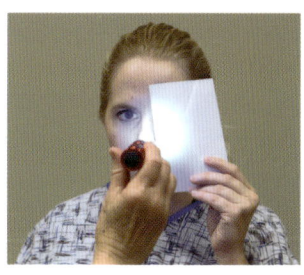

Direct and indirect pupillary reaction to light.

- **Accommodation:** Hold your finger about 6 inches from the patient's face, and ask the patient to look back and forth from your finger to a distant object. Watch for pupillary size change as the patient looks back and forth from your finger to a distant object.

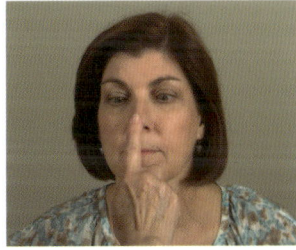

Accommodation and Convergence.

- **Convergence:** Ask the patient to maintain focus on your finger as you move it from 6 inches in front of her face to the tip of her nose. Watch for eyes to converge, or "cross" medially.
- Assess for ptosis (lid lag) during eye movements.

Expected Report

- Pupils are 3 mm and equal in size; pupils react equally to direct and indirect light.
- Pupils constrict and dilate in response to focus on far and near objects.
- Eyes converge bilaterally to focus on a near object.
- There is no ptosis.
- Note that PERRLA (abbreviation for "pupils equal, round, reactive to light and accommodation") or a similar abbreviation is often used to indicate the assessment findings related to the pupils.

Benign Variations

- Pupil size may be 2 mm to 9 mm and varies with the degree of light and emotions.
  - Heredity influences pupil size.
- Note that the pupillary light reflex also tests CN II, Optic.

Unexpected Findings: See p. 168.

HEENT

CN III, Oculomotor; CN IV, Trochlear; CN VI, Abducens

Inspection

- Extraocular eye movements (EOMs) are controlled by the 6 extraocular muscles and the integrated actions of CNs III, IV, and VI.
  - Movements should be smooth and symmetrical without nystagmus (jerky eye movements).
- To assess CNs III, IV, and VI extraocular muscle innervation functions, stand in front of the patient.
- Ask the patient to follow your finger visually without moving his head as you move your finger through the 6 cardinal fields of gaze. These are:
  1. **Right superior gaze**—Tests CN III, Oculomotor, Superior rectus muscle (right eye) and Inferior oblique muscle (left eye)
  2. **Left superior gaze**—Tests CN III, Oculomotor, Superior rectus muscle (left eye) and Inferior oblique muscle (right eye)
  3. **Left lateral gaze**—Tests CN III, Oculomotor, Lateral rectus muscle (left eye) and CN VI, Abducens, Medial rectus muscle (right eye)
  4. **Left inferior gaze**—Tests CN III, Oculomotor, Inferior rectus muscle (left eye) and CN IV, Trochlear, Superior oblique muscle (right eye)
  5. **Right inferior gaze**—Tests CN III, Oculomotor, Inferior rectus muscle (right eye) and CN IV, Trochlear, Superior oblique muscle (left eye)
  6. **Right lateral gaze**—Tests CN III, Oculomotor, Lateral rectus muscle (right eye) and CN VI, Abducens, Medial rectus muscle (left eye)

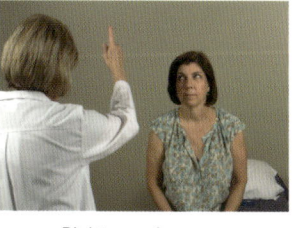

Right superior gaze.

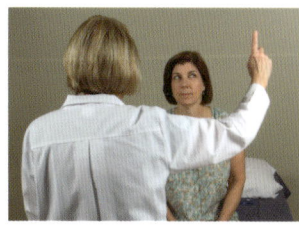

Left superior gaze.

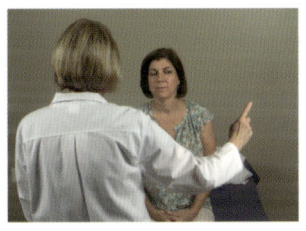

Left lateral gaze.

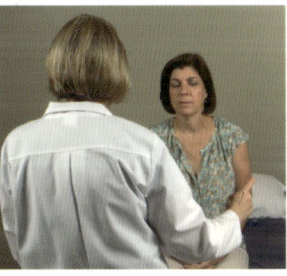

Left inferior gaze.

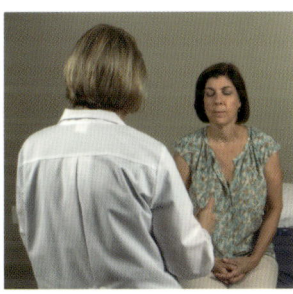

Right inferior gaze.

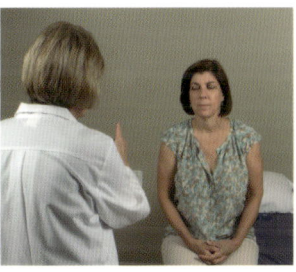

Right lateral gaze.

Expected Report
- Eyes move in a coordinated fashion through the 6 cardinal fields of gaze without nystagmus
- CN III, Oculomotor, IV, Trochlear, and VI, Oculomotor intact

Benign Variations
- A few beats of nystagmus (jerky eye movements) may be seen with extreme lateral gaze.

Unexpected Findings: See p. 168.

HEENT

CN II, Optic

Visual Acuity—Distant Vision

■ Assess far vision using a Snellen chart or other standard chart.
■ Ask patient to stand 20 ft. from the Snellen chart and:
  ■ Cover left eye with a card or other object, and use the right eye to read lowest line possible.
  ■ Cover right eye, and assess the left eye in the same manner.
  ■ With both eyes uncovered, read the lowest line possible. This is known as *binocular vision*.
    • If patient wears corrective lenses, vision is usually assessed with patient wearing them.
    • Note that the top number in 20/20 or 20/40, etc., is the number of feet between the patient and the eye chart. If distant vision is assessed in a small room or area, the patient may stand 10 feet from the chart, resulting in the top number being 10 rather than 20.
    • The bottom number in 20/20 or 20/40, etc., is the number found on the chart row of the smallest print that the patient can read. The bottom number represents the distance (in feet) at which the "normal" eye can read the letters on that line.

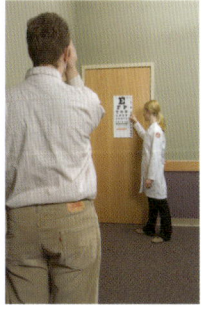

Distant vision using Snellen chart (Dillon, P. (2007). *Nursing health assessment: A critical thinking case studies approach* (2 ed.). Philadelphia: F. A. Davis Company.)

Visual Acuity—Near Vision

- Assess near vision by asking patient to read a newspaper or Rosenbaum chart
- Hold or ask the patient to hold printed material about 14" from patient's eyes
  - Assess one eye at a time.
  - Assess both eyes at the same time.
  - If patient wears corrective lenses, assess with patient wearing lenses

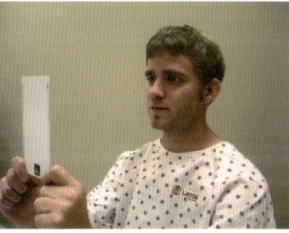

Near vision.

Expected Report (Distant and Near Vision)

- Distant vision 20/20 bilaterally in each eye and with binocular vision
- Reads newsprint with the paper held approximately 14" from the eyes
- CN II, Optic, distant and near vision intact

Benign Variations

- If corrected lenses are worn while distant vision is assessed, findings should be "Vision 20/20 with corrective lenses."
- As patient ages, the lens of the eye becomes less elastic, and the ability to focus on near objects without the use of corrective lenses diminishes.
- If corrective lenses are worn during near vision assessment, record the strength of the lenses, such as "Reads newsprint accurately with +2.0 corrective lenses."

Unexpected Findings: See p. 168.

Confrontation Test

- Assess peripheral vision or "visual fields" via the confrontation test.
- To perform the confrontation test:
  1. The examiner stands directly in front of the patient.
  2. Ask the patient to cover the right eye with a card or hand while you cover your left eye.

3. Ask the patient to look directly at your nose and tell you when she sees your wiggling fingers as you slowly bring your fingers toward the center from the upper right, upper left, lower right, and lower left as well as from above and then below your field of vision.

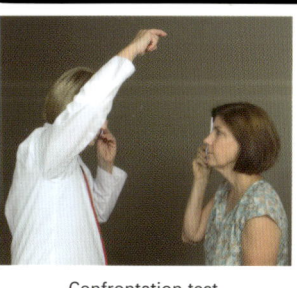

Confrontation test.

Expected Report

■ Visual fields equal to those of the examiner

■ Cranial Nerve II, Optic, peripheral vision intact

Unexpected Findings: See p. 168.

Retinal or Fundoscopic Exam

■ Dim the lights in the room to encourage pupillary dilation.

■ Ask the patient to look over your left shoulder and stare at a fixed object several feet away.

■ Place your left hand on the patient's head to prevent movement, and use you left thumb to gently lift and immobilize the patient's right eyelid.

   ■ *Note that in some cultures, touching another person's head is regarded as disrespectful, so first ask for permission.*

■ Use an ophthalmoscope held in your right hand, in front of your right eye and braced against your right eyebrow, to assess the retina of the patient's right eye.

■ Note the red reflex that appears as an orange glow in the pupil as you shine the light toward the eye.

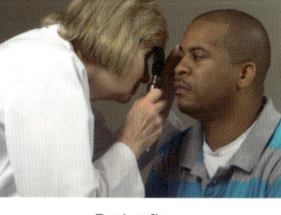

   ■ The red reflex is best seen at about 15 inches from the patient's eye and about 15 degrees lateral to the eye.

■ Assess the lens for opacities (cataracts).

Red reflex.

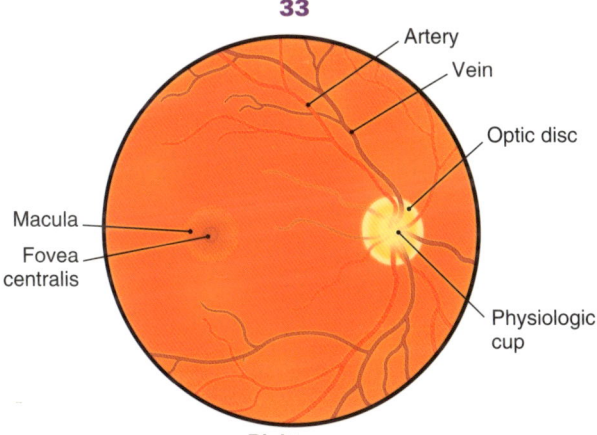

Artery

Vein

Optic disc

Macula

Fovea
centralis

Physiologic
cup

Right eye

Retina (Dillon, P. (2007). *Nursing health assessment: A critical thinking case studies approach.* (2 ed.). Philadelphia: F. A. Davis Company.)

- Keeping the red reflex in view, move slowly toward the patient's right eye until the ophthalmoscope touches your thumb that is supporting the patient's upper right eyelid.
- Locate the circular-shaped optic disk by following the path of a retinal blood vessel nasally to the place where it converges with other vessels at the optic disk.
- Use the adjustable wheel on the ophthalmoscope to focus on the optic disk.
- Assess the optic disk and cup for:
  - Color
  - Appearance and clarity of disk margins
  - Elevation
  - Cup:disk ratio
    - Cup:disk ratio should be less than 1:2 or may be stated as less than 0.5.

- Follow arterioles and venules from the optic disk in 4 different directions to assess for vessel damage and retinal lesions.
- Compare the color and relative size of the arterioles and venules.
  - Note that arterioles are smaller and more brightly red colored than venules.
- Note presence of:
  - Nicking at vessel crossings, called AV nicking
  - Hemorrhages
  - Copper wiring
  - Cotton wool
  - Exudates
- Direct your light beam laterally from the optic disk, or ask the patient to look directly into the light to assess the fovea and the surrounding macula.
  - A bright reflection is expected, and the patient generally indicates discomfort as the macula is the retina's area of "central vision," meaning that it is used to look directly at an object, rather than for "peripheral vision."
- Examine the left eye in the same manner, using your right hand to steady the patient's head and your right thumb to lift the eyelid.

Expected Report
- The red reflex is present in both eyes.
- The optic disks are yellowish orange with clear margins and no apparent swelling or elevation.
- The cup: disk ratio is less than 1:2.
- Arterioles are brighter and smaller than venules, with a ratio of 2:3.
- No AV nicking, hemorrhages, copper wiring, cotton wool, or exudates are seen on the retinal blood vessels.
- The macula is noted about two disk diameters from the optic disk.

Benign Variations
- The optic disk may be creamy pink.

Unexpected Findings: See pp. 168–169.

Assessing the Nose

Inspection

- Inspect external nose for symmetry
- Use a gloved hand to lift the tip of the nose upward as you look inside the nose to inspect the nasal septum for:
  - Deviation
  - Intactness
  - Color of the nasal mucosa
  - Nasal mucus:
    - Amount
    - Color
    - Consistency
- Inspect the nasal passages for:
  - Patency
  - Swollen turbinates
  - Redness of turbinates
    - Turbinates normally look like the fingers of a glove, with one appearing to be stacked behind the other when the inside walls of the nares are visualized.
  - Polyps
- Assess for bilateral nasal patency by having patient inhale while occluding one naris and then the other

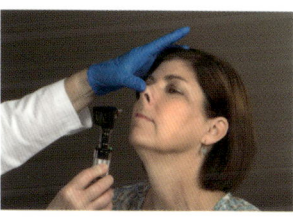

Inspect nasal septum and passages.

Expected Report

- Nose symmetrical in shape with septum midline and intact
- Nasal mucosa pink; scant amount of thin, clear mucus observed
- Nasal passages bilaterally patent
- No visible redness or swelling of the turbinates and no visible polyps; air moves into and out of each nostril during respirations

Benign Variations

- Nose and/or septum may be slightly asymmetrical

Unexpected Findings: See p. 169.

CN I, Olfactory

Sensory Function
- Assess sense of smell.
- Ask patient to close eyes and alternately occlude each naris individually while you hold an object with a familiar odor (such as coffee, vanilla, or peppermint) below the nose.
  - A different odor should be used to assess sense of smell in each nares.

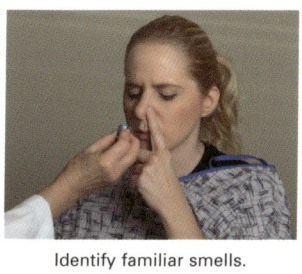

Identify familiar smells.

Expected Report
- Identifies familiar smells
- Cranial nerve I, Olfactory intact

Unexpected Findings: *See p. 169.*

Assessing the Sinuses

Inspection
- Ask patient to open his mouth.
- Transilluminate sinuses by placing the tip of your penlight or otoscope light against the patient's face in the area over the maxillary sinuses as you look into the mouth.
  - Light should be seen in mouth.

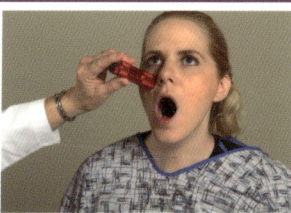

Sinus transillumination.

Palpation

- Assess for pain by pushing with your thumb tips over the maxillary sinuses.
- Tap lightly over the frontal sinuses.

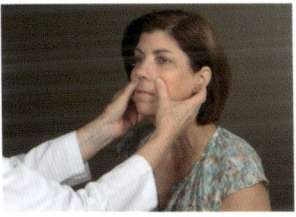

Palpate over maxillary sinuses.

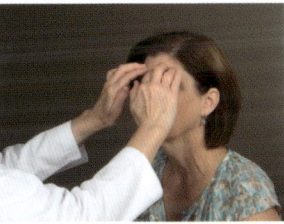

Tap over frontal sinuses.

Expected Report

- Light clearly seen in the mouth with transillumination of maxillary sinuses
- No tenderness noted over maxillary or frontal sinuses

Unexpected Findings: See p. 169.

Assessing the Mouth

Assessing the Lips

Inspection

- Inspect the lips for:
  - Color
  - Moistness
  - Cracking
  - Lesions

Expected Report

- Lips pink and moist without cracking or lesions

Unexpected Findings: See p. 170.

HEENT

Assessing the Teeth

Inspection
- Assess teeth:
  - Number
  - Alignment
  - Condition
- Ask patient to close mouth and show you his teeth
- Inspect bite alignment

Expected Report
- There are 32 tight-fitting teeth without caries or restorations.
- Front teeth align without signs of underbite or overbite.

Benign Variations
- Fewer than 32 teeth may be genetic but is more commonly caused by tooth extraction related to crowding, severe caries, or infection
- Restorations with amalgam or other type fillings or dental crowns over partial teeth are common in older patients who were children before fluoride was added to toothpastes and public drinking water

Unexpected Findings: See p. 170.

Assessing the Oral Mucosa and Gums

Inspection
- Don nonsterile gloves.
- Ask patient to open his mouth.
- Inspect the oral mucosa for:
  - Color
  - Intactness
  - Lesions
- Use a tongue blade to assist with inspection of:
  - Mucosa near the gumline
  - Buccal mucosa
- Inspect the gums for:
  - Color
  - Lesions

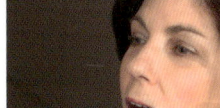

Inspect lips and mucous membranes.

38

- Erosion (receding)
- Bleeding

Expected Report
- Oral mucosa pink and intact without lesions
- Gums pink without lesions or signs of receding, irritation, or bleeding

Benign Variations
- It is normal for dark-skinned people to have bluish mucous membranes.

Unexpected Findings: See p. 170.

Assessing the Salivary Glands

Inspection
- Inspect the salivary glands for swelling and tumors.
- Salivary glands are:
  - Parotid gland
  - Submandibular gland
  - Sublingual gland

Expected Report
- No swelling or tumors of salivary glands noted

Unexpected Findings: See p. 170.

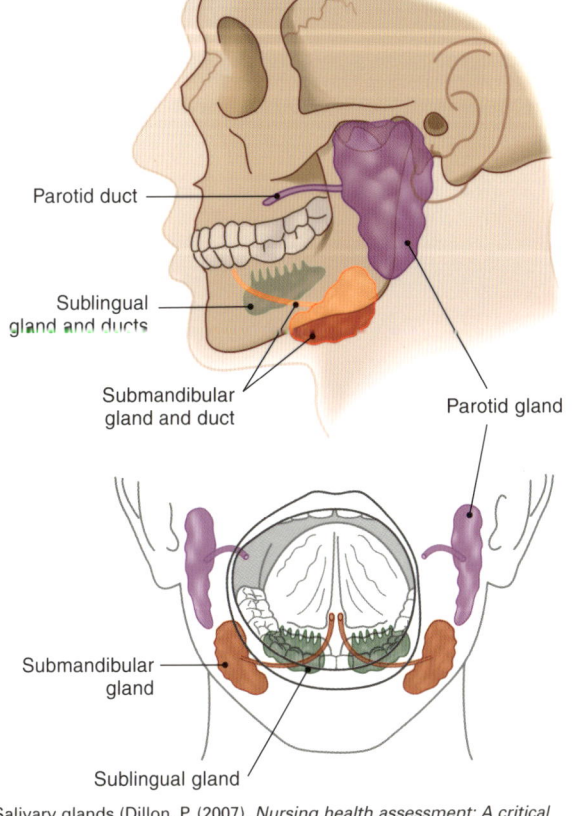

Parotid duct

Sublingual gland and ducts

Submandibular gland and duct

Parotid gland

Submandibular gland

Sublingual gland

Salivary glands (Dillon, P. (2007). *Nursing health assessment: A critical thinking case studies approach.* (2 ed.). Philadelphia: F. A. Davis Company.)

Assessing the Tongue

Inspection
- Use a tongue blade or gloved fingers to lift the tongue.
- Inspect ventral (bottom), dorsal (top), and lateral (side) surfaces of the tongue for:
  - Moistness
  - Lesions
  - Coating

Expected Report
- Tongue moist
- No lesions or coating seen on ventral, dorsal, or lateral surfaces

Benign Variations
- *Geographic tongue* is a benign condition in which patches on the surface of the tongue are missing papillae and may appear as slightly raised and reddened areas.

Unexpected Findings: See p. 170

Assess the Pharynx and Tonsils

Inspection
- Inspect hard and soft palates for intactness and continuity.
- Inspect pharynx for:
  - Color
  - Postnasal drainage
  - Lesions
- Inspect tonsils for:
  - Size
  - Color
  - Exudate

Expected Report
- Hard and soft palates intact and continuous
- Pharynx pink with postnasal drainage lesions
- Tonsils small and pink without exudate

Benign Variations
- ■ Tonsils may be absent due to surgical removal.
- ■ Irregular indentions (crypts) may be seen on surface of tonsils.

Unexpected Findings: See p. 171.

CN XII, Hypoglossal

Inspection
- ■ Inspect tongue for:
  - ■ Symmetry
  - ■ Tremors
- ■ Ask patient to stick out tongue and move it side to side as you resist movement with the side of a tongue blade
- ■ Evaluate speech for clarity during conversation
  - ■ Note that CN XII is one of several CNs that contribute to clear enunciation of words.

Tongue symmetry.

Tongue strength.

Expected Report
- ■ Tongue is symmetrical and without tremors
- ■ There is strong resistance to tongue movement with a tongue blade
- ■ Clearly enunciates words
- ■ Cranial nerve XII intact

Unexpected Findings: See p. 170.

CN IX, Glossopharyngeal
CN X, Vagus

- Assess ability to identify sour (posterior lateral portion of tongue) and bitter (back of tongue) tastes.
- Assess the gag reflex by lightly touching the back of the pharynx with a tongue blade to test CN IX, Glossopharyngeal, sensory function and CN X, Vagus, motor function.
- Ask the patient to swallow as you observe for difficulty swallowing CN IX, Glossopharyngeal, sensory function and CN X, Vagus, motor function.
- Ask the patient to say "ahh" as you observe for symmetrical movement of the uvula and for hoarseness to test CN X, Vagus.

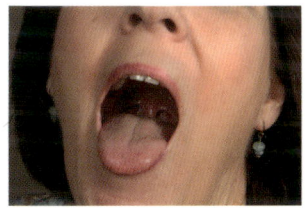

Uvula rises midline.

Expected Report
- Patient identifies both sour and bitter tastes, CN IX, Glossopharyngeal intact
- Gag reflex intact, CN IX, Glossopharyngeal, sensory function and CN X, Vagus, motor function, intact
- Swallows with ease, CN IX, Glossopharyngeal, sensory function and CN X, Vagus, motor function, intact
- Uvula rises in midline, and there is no hoarseness as the patient vocalizes the "ahh" sound

Unexpected Findings: See p. 171

Assessing the Ear

Assessing the Outer Ear

Inspection

■ Inspect outer ears for placement and lesions

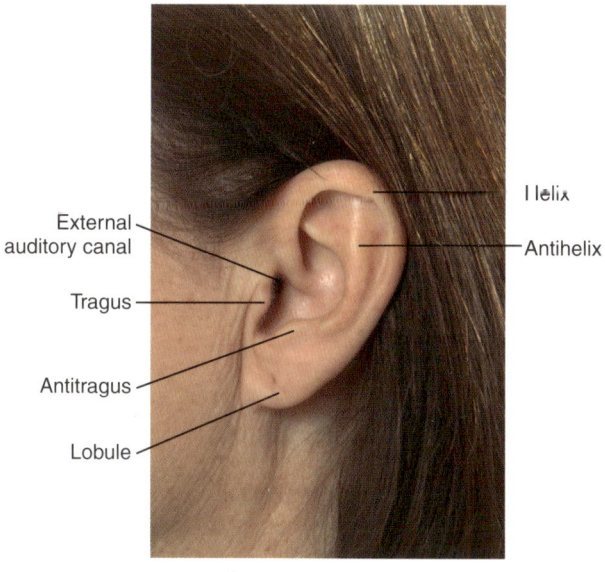

External
auditory canal

Tragus

Antitragus

Lobule

Helix

Antihelix

Inspect outer ear.

Palpation

■ Palpate outer ear structures for tenderness and masses.

Expected Report
- Tops of ears in alignment with inner canthus of eyes
- No lesions seen on external ears
- No complaints of tenderness with palpation of outer ear structures

Unexpected Findings: See p. 171.

CN VIII, Vestibulocochlear or Acoustic

- CN VIII has two sensory functions:
  1. Hearing
  2. Vestibular function
     - Vestibular system sends information to the brain to help maintain balance

Gross Hearing, Whisper Test

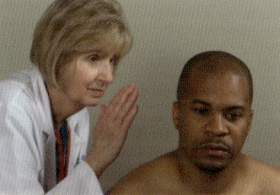

- Stand about 12 inches behind patient
- Ask patient to occlude one ear canal
- Whisper a two-syllable word such as "baseball," and ask patient to identify the word
- Repeat the test on the opposite ear, using different word

Whisper test.

Expected Report
- Identifies whispered words

Unexpected Findings: See p. 171.

Weber Test

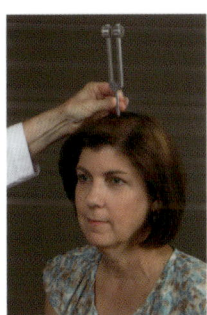

- Activate a 512- or 256-Hz tuning fork, and place it on top of the patient's head or on the patient's forehead.
- Ask patient, "Please tell me if you hear the sound better in one ear than the other or if you hear it equally in both ears."

Expected Report
- Hears sound equally in both ears

Unexpected Findings: See p. 171.

Weber test.

Rinne Test

- Activate a tuning fork, and place the handle tip on the mastoid bone, just behind the auricle of one ear.
- Ask patient, "Please tell me when you stop hearing the sound."
- After patient stops hearing the sound, hold the tuning fork in front of the auricle of the ear, and say, "Tell me when the sounds stops."
  - Note the tuning fork is *not* reactivated when it is moved from the mastoid process and placed in front of the ear auricle.

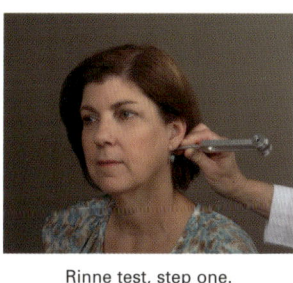
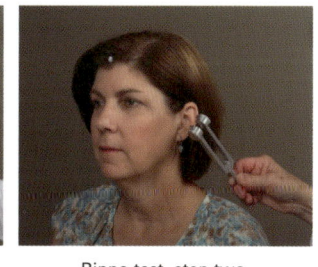

Rinne test, step one.   Rinne test, step two.

Expected Report

- Air conduction approximately twice as long as bone conduction
- Cranial nerve VIII, Acoustic, hearing component intact

Unexpected Findings: See p. 171.

Vestibular Test

- Place your hands on the side of the patient's head, and turn his head from side to side as you watch the direction of his gaze (doll's eye maneuver).

Expected Report

- Eye focus moves to the right as patient's head is turned to the left, and focus moves to the left as head is turned to the right

Unexpected Findings: See p. 171.

Assessing the Ear Canal

Inspection
- Use lighted otoscope to inspect ear canal for:
  - Patency
  - Color
  - Cerumen
  - Foreign bodies
  - Drainage

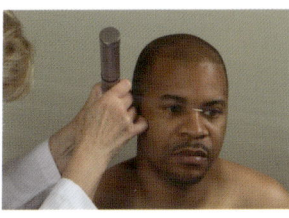

Otoscopic exam.

Expected Report
- Ear canals patent and pink without swelling, excess cerumen, foreign bodies, or drainage.

Unexpected Findings: See p. 172.

Assessing the Tympanic Membrane

Inspection
- Use lighted otoscope to inspect tympanic membrane (TM) for:
  - Intactness
  - Color
  - Light reflex
  - Retraction or bulging
  - Bony structures

  Note: Light reflex should be an uninterrupted triangular-shaped reflection of the otoscope's light; it should point toward the face and widen toward the center of the TM.

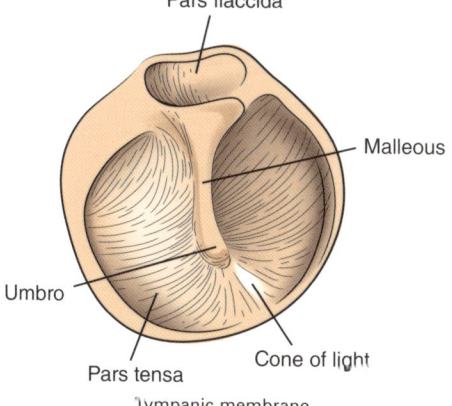

Pars flaccida

Malleous

Umbro

Cone of light

Pars tensa

Tympanic membrane.

Expected Report

■ TM is intact and pearly gray in color with an uninterrupted light reflex at 7 o'clock in the left ear and at 5 o'clock in the right ear
■ No bulging or retraction of the TM noted
■ Bony landmarks are intact, with the umbo appearing near the center of the TM

Benign Variations

■ Crying may cause the TM to appear red.

Unexpected Findings: See p. 172.

CN XI, Spinal Accessory

CN XI innervates the sternocleidomastoid and the trapezius muscles.

Inspection

■ Ask patient to shrug his shoulders as you push downward on the tops of his shoulders.
■ Ask patient to turn his head from side to side as you provide resistance to turning by holding the palm of your hand against the side of his face.

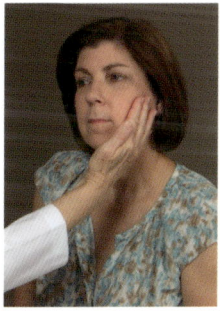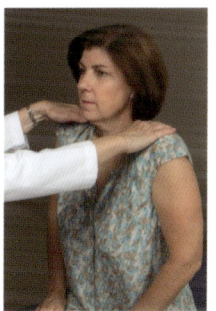

Turn head against resistance.

Shrug shoulders.

Expected Report
- Shrugs shoulders against resistance
- Turns face from side to side against resistance
- CN XI, Spinal Accessory, intact

Unexpected Findings: See p. 172.

Assessing the Neck

Assessing the Lymph Nodes of the Head and Neck

Inspection
- Inspect lymph nodes for:
  - Size
  - Redness

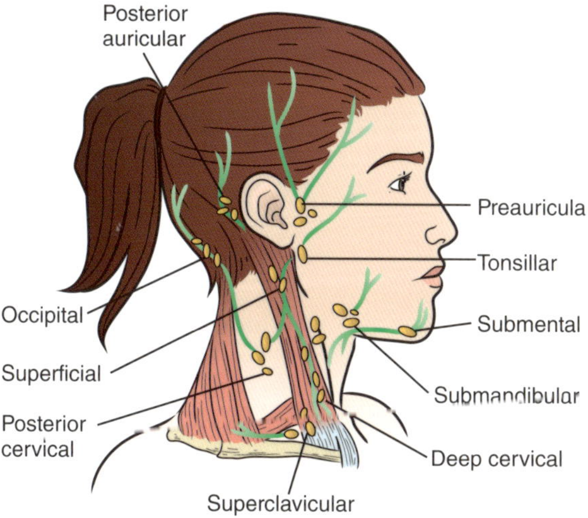

Posterior
auricular

Preauricula

Tonsillar

Occipital

Submental

Superficial

Submandibular

Posterior
cervical

Deep cervical

Superclavicular

Lymph nodes of the head and neck.

Palpation

■ Palpate lymph nodes using a circular
motion with your fingertips for:
  ■ Size
  ■ Tenderness
  ■ Mobility
    • Assess the following lymph nodes as
      noted in illustration:
      – Preauricular   – Submandibular
      – Postauricular   – Submental
      – Occipital   – Tonsillar
      – Cervical   – Posterior cervical
      – Deep   – Supraclavicular
      – Superficial

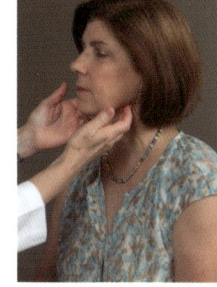

Palpate lymph nodes.

Expected Report
- Lymph nodes of head and neck are non-tender and nonpalpable.

Benign Variations
- "Shotty" nodes are hard, mobile, and about the size of birdshot or BB gun ammunition. They may be the result of past infections.

Unexpected Findings: See p. 172.

Assessing the Thyroid

Inspection
- Inspect thyroid area for:
  - Enlargement
  - Masses
- Ask the patient to swallow a sip of water while assessing for upward movement of the thyroid gland.
  - Note that tangential lighting may reveal unnoticed irregularities.

Palpation
- Palpate thyroid for:
  - Tenderness
  - Masses
  - Palpate standing in front of the patient and standing behind the patient

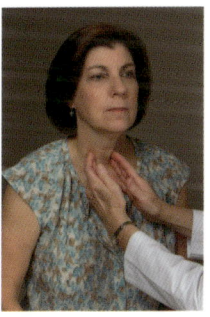 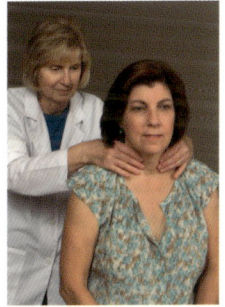

Anterior thyroid palpation. Posterior thyroid palpation.

HEENT

Expected Report

■ No enlargement or masses visible in the thyroid area
■ Thyroid tissue is smooth and non-tender to palpation and without palpable masses

Unexpected Findings: See p. 172.

HEENT Assessment Check-Off List

Assessment Task	Performed and Reported Correctly	Performed or Reported Incorrectly	Not Performed
HEAD			
Head, size and shape			
Head, symmetry			
Head, lumps and bumps			
Head, tenderness			
Head, lesions, scars			
Head, scaling			
Head, parasitic infestation			
FACE			
Facial feature symmetry			
Facial expression			
CN V, Trigeminal, motor, bite strength & symmetry			
CNV, Trigeminal, sensory, facial, touch, and blink reflex			
CN VII, Facial, motor, make faces			
EYES			
Eyebrows, quantity			
Eyebrows, placement			
Eyebrows, color			
Eyelashes, direction, distal tips, entropion, ectropion			

HEENT Assessment Check-Off List—cont'd

Assessment Task	Performed and Reported Correctly	Performed or Reported Incorrectly	Not Performed
Eyelid position relative to eye structures, ptosis			
Eyelid, lesions			
Lacrimal apparatus, swelling			
Lacrimal apparatus, redness			
Lacrimal apparatus, drainage			
Lacrimal apparatus, tenderness			
Globe of eye, protrusion			
Conjunctiva, color			
Conjunctive, moisture			
Sclera, color			
Iris, color			
Iris, shape			
Cornea, transparency			
Corneal light reflex			
Cover-uncover test			
Pupil size			
CN III, Oculomotor, direct pupillary light reflex			
CN III, Oculomotor, indirect pupillary light reflex			
Pupil accommodation			
Pupil convergence			
Ptosis			
CN III, Oculomotor, CN IV, Trochlear, CN VI, Abducens, extraocular eye movements, 6 cardinal fields of gaze			

Continued

HEENT

HEENT Assessment Check-Off List—cont'd

Assessment Task	Performed and Reported Correctly	Performed or Reported Incorrectly	Not Performed
Nystagmus			
Distant vision			
Near vision			
Confrontation test			
Red reflex			
Lens, opacities (cataracts)			
Optic disk and cup, color			
Optic disk and cup, clarity of disk margins			
Optic disk and cup, elevation			
Optic disk and cup, disk ratio			
Arteriole to venule color and size comparison			
Vessel, nicking			
Vessel, hemorrhages			
Vessel, copper wiring			
Vessel, cotton wool			
Vessel, exudates			
Macula			
NOSE			
Nose, symmetry			
Septum, deviation			
Septum, intactness			
Nasal passage, patency			
Mucosa, color			
Mucus, amount			
Mucus, color			
Mucus, consistency			
Turbinates, swelling			

HEENT Assessment Check-Off List—cont'd

Assessment Task	Performed and Reported Correctly	Performed or Reported Incorrectly	Not Performed
Turbinates, redness			
Polyps			
CN I, Olfactory, sense of smell			
SINUSES			
Sinus transillumination			
Sinus, palpation & tap			
MOUTH			
Lips, color			
Lips, moistness			
Lips, cracking			
Lips, lesions			
Teeth, number			
Teeth, alignment			
Teeth, condition			
Bite alignment			
Oral mucosa, color			
Oral mucosa, intactness			
Oral mucosa, lesions			
Gums, color			
Gums, lesions			
Gums, erosion			
Gums, bleeding			
Salivary gland, parotid, swelling			
Salivary gland, submandibular, swelling			
Salivary gland, sublingual, swelling			

Continued

HEENT

HEENT Assessment Check-Off List—cont'd

Assessment Task	Performed and Reported Correctly	Performed or Reported Incorrectly	Not Performed
Tongue, moistness			
Tongue, lesions			
Tongue, coating			
Hard and soft palate			
Pharynx, color			
Pharynx, postnasal drainage			
Pharynx, lesions			
Tonsils, size			
Tonsils, color			
Tonsils, exudate			
Tongue, symmetry			
Tongue, tremors			
CN IX, Glossopharyngeal, taste			
Gag reflex, CN IX, Glossopharyngeal, for sensory and CN X, Vagus, for motor gag reflex			
Swallow, CN IX, Glossopharyngeal, for sensory and CN X, Vagus, for motor			
CN X, uvula rises midline			
CN IX and CN X, hoarseness			
EAR			
Outer ear, placement			
Outer ear, lesions			
Outer ear, tenderness			
Outer ear, masses			
Ear canal, patency			

HEENT Assessment Check-Off List—cont'd			
Assessment Task	Performed and Reported Correctly	Performed or Reported Incorrectly	Not Performed
Ear canal, color			
Ear canal, cerumen			
Ear canal, foreign bodies			
Ear canal, drainage			
CN VIII, Vestibulocochlear, Acoustic, identify whispered words			
CN VIII, Acoustic, Weber test, two steps			
CN VIII, Acoustic, Rinne test, two steps			
CN VIII, Vestibular, doll's eye maneuver			
Tympanic membrane, intactness			
Tympanic membrane, color			
Tympanic membrane, light reflex			
Tympanic membrane, retraction or bulging			
Tympanic membrane, bony structures			
CN XI, Spinal accessory, shrug shoulders			
CN XI, Spinal accessory, turn head, side to side against resistance			
Pre-auricular lymph nodes, observe and palpate			
Postauricular			

Continued

HEENT

HEENT Assessment Check-Off List—cont'd

Assessment Task	Performed and Reported Correctly	Performed or Reported Incorrectly	Not Performed
Occipital lymph nodes, observe and palpate			
Cervical lymph nodes, observe and palpate deep and superficial nodes			
Submandibular lymph nodes, observe and palpate			
Submental lymph nodes, observe and palpate			
Tonsillar			
Posterior cervical			
Supraclavicular			
THYROID			
Thyroid, visualize for size & masses			
Thyroid, anterior palpation for tenderness, enlargement & masses			
Thyroid, posterior palpation for tenderness, enlargement & masses			

Preparing for the Chest and Breast Assessment

Gather Equipment
- Stethoscope
- Small pillow (optional)
- Small ruler with mm and cm markings
- Felt-tip pen
- Percussion hammer (optional)

Prepare Patient
- Explain the procedure.
- Ask the patient to sit upright with his arms at his side.
- Clothes should be removed and a drape provided.

Examiner
- Stand in front of the patient for the anterior and lateral chest assessment.
- Stand behind the patient for the posterior chest assessment.

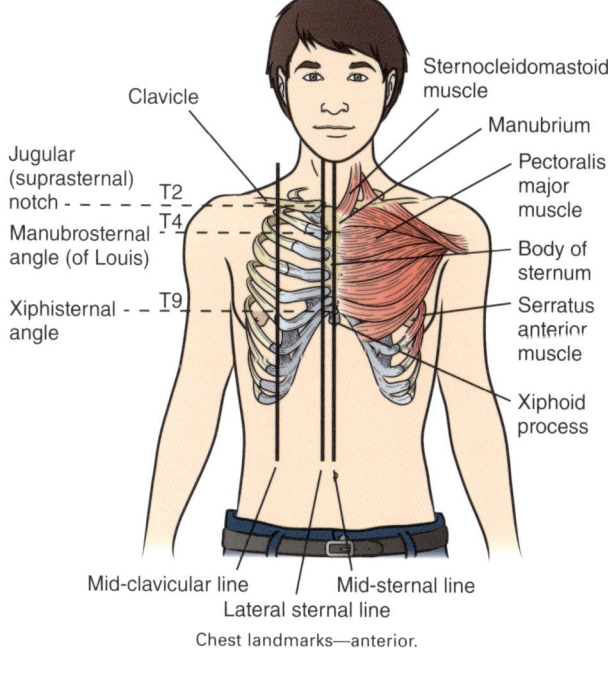

Clavicle

Sternocleidomastoid
muscle

Manubrium

Pectoralis
major
muscle

Jugular
(suprasternal)
notch

T2

T4

Manubrosternal
angle (of Louis)

Body of
sternum

Xiphisternal
angle

T9

Serratus
anterior
muscle

Xiphoid
process

Mid-clavicular line

Mid-sternal line

Lateral sternal line

Chest landmarks—anterior.

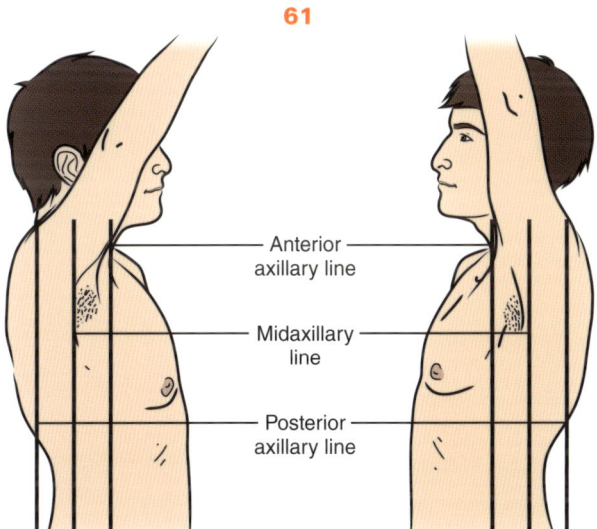

Anterior axillary line

Midaxillary line

Posterior axillary line

Chest landmarks—lateral.

Lungs.

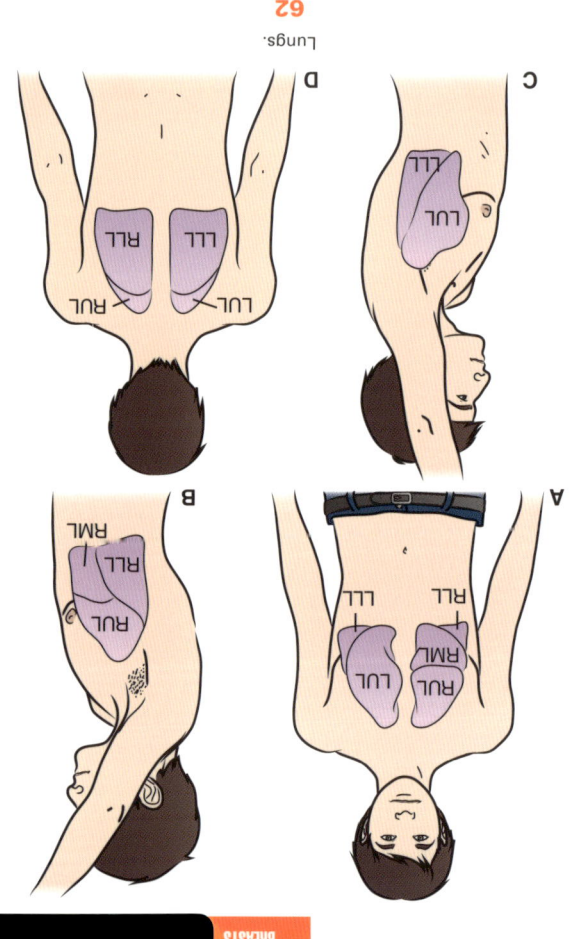

Assessing the Chest

Assessing the Anterior and Axillary Chest

Inspection

- Inspect the anterior and axillary chest for:
  - Lesions
  - Scars
  - Deformities
  - Symmetry, including symmetrical rise and fall of chest during respirations
- Compare anteroposterior with lateral chest diameter; this is commonly called the AP ratio.
- Observe respiratory:
  - Rate
  - Rhythm or pattern
  - Effort
- Estimate the costal angle, also known as substernal or infrasternal angle

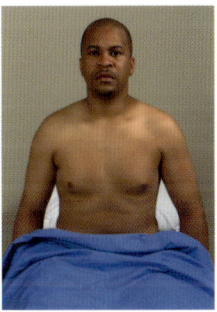

Inspect anterior chest.

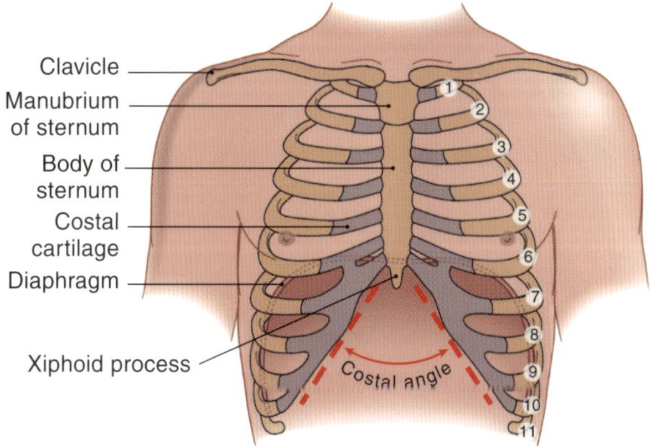

Clavicle
Manubrium of sternum
Body of sternum
Costal cartilage
Diaphragm
Xiphoid process
Costal angle
1
2
3
4
5
6
7
8
9
10
11

Costal angle (Dillon, P. (2007). *Nursing health assessment: A critical thinking case studies approach* (2nd ed.). Philadelphia: F.A. Davis Company.)

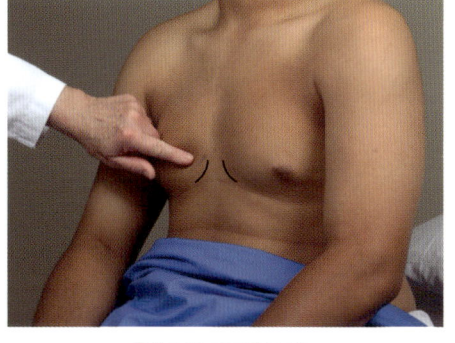

Estimate costal angle.

Expected Report
- The anterior chest is symmetrical and without lesions, scars, or deformities.
- There is symmetrical rise and fall of the chest during respirations.
- The anteroposterior to lateral chest diameter ratio is 1:2.
- The respiratory rate is 14 breaths per minute.
- Respirations are even, quiet, and unlabored.
- The costal angle is less than 90°.

Benign Variations
- The AP diameter generally increases with age; e.g., the chest appears more rounded.
- Spinal kyphosis may cause the chest to appear more rounded.
- The sustained respiratory rate may be 12 to 20 breaths per minute in the adult and may be slower or faster for brief periods.

Unexpected Findings: See pp. 172–173.

Palpation
- Palpate the anterior and axillary chest for:
    - Masses
    - Complaints of discomfort
    - Crepitus
- Place the palms of your open hands over the right and left superior anterior lung fields.
- Ask the patient to say "99" as move your hands inferiorly to assess bilaterally the quality of tactile fremitus and compare the vibrations felt in the right and left lung fields.
    - Tactile fremitus is the palpable vibration of the chest wall produced by speech.
- Assess anterior respiratory excursion by placing your open hands on each side of the patient's lower rib cage in the axillary lines, and ask the patient to inhale deeply and then exhale.
    - Watch for symmetrical movement as your hands move laterally with inspiration and medially with expiration.

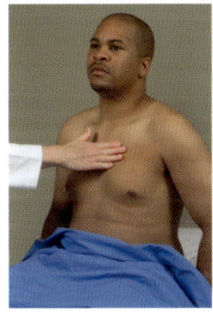

Palpate anterior chest and assess fremitus.

Expected Report

- No masses, crepitus, or complaints of discomfort with palpation of the anterior and axillary chest
- Moderate vibration is felt equally throughout the chest wall as the patient says "99."
  - Note vibration may be slightly less over inferior lungs fields

Unexpected Findings: See p. 173.

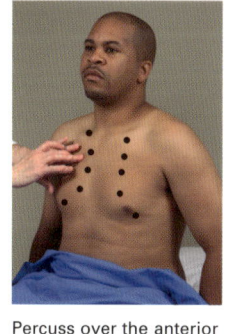

Percuss over the anterior and axillary airways.

Percussion

- Use indirect percussion to assess bilaterally the percussion tone over the anterior and axillary airways and lung fields.

Expected Report

- There is resonance to percussion throughout the anterior and axillary airways and lung fields, with dullness heard over the precordium and liver.

Unexpected Findings: See p. 173.

Auscultation

- Use the diaphragm of the stethoscope to auscultate over the anterior and axillary lung fields as you move the stethoscope to compare sounds over the right and left lung fields.
  - Note that breath sounds in the right middle lobe are heard best between the 4th and 6th ribs in the right axilla.
- Note:
  - Location of auscultation
  - Pitch of sound
  - Comparison of inspiratory and expiratory duration
  - Adventitious sounds
    - **Rales**: Crackling sound similar to that of dry leaves rubbed between your fingers
      - Rales may also be called crackles.
      - Rales are most often heard with inspiration and in the lower lobes.

– There are other subtypes of rales:
  - **Wheeze:** Musical, high pitched sounds may be called musical rales or sibilant rhonchi; wheezes can be inspiratory, expiratory, or both
  - **Rhonchi:** Low-pitched, coarse, or snoring-like sounds that may clear after the patient coughs

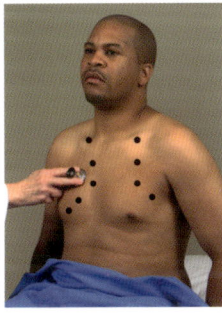

| Auscultate anterior lung fields. | Auscultate right middle lobe. |

Expected Report
- High-pitched bronchial breath sounds are heard over the trachea, with expiration lasting longer than inspiration.
- Medium-pitched bronchovesicular breath sounds are heard over the main bronchus, with expiration and inspiration being equal in duration.
- Low-pitched vesicular sounds are heard throughout the peripheral lungs fields, with inspiration lasting longer than expiration.
- No crackles, wheezes, or rhonchi heard.

Unexpected Findings: See p. 174.

Assessing the Posterior Chest

Inspection
- Stand behind the patient to assess the posterior chest.
- Inspect posterior chest for:
  - Lesions
  - Scars
  - Deformities
  - Symmetry, including symmetry of chest movement during respirations
- Inspect spinal alignment and natural spinal curves.

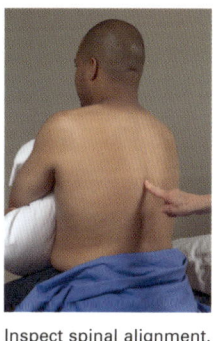

Inspect spinal alignment.

Expected Report
- There are no lesions, scars, or deformities of the posterior chest.
- The posterior chest is symmetrical with symmetrical respiratory movements.
- The spine is midline and slightly concave in the cervical area, slightly convex in the thoracic area, and slightly concave in the lumbar area.
  - Note that spinal alignment and curves may be assessed during the MS assessment.

Unexpected Findings: See p. 174.

Palpation
- Palpate the posterior chest for:
  - Masses
  - Discomfort
- Place your thumbs near the spine as your open hands rest on the lower rib cage. Observe for symmetrical respiratory excursion as the patient inhales and exhales.
- Lightly place the palms of your hands over the right and left superior lung fields.
- Ask the patient to say "99" as you move your hands inferiorly over all the posterior airways to assess tactile fremitus.

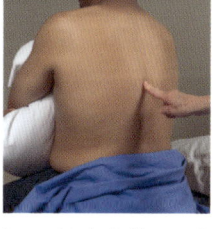

Palpation of posterior chest.

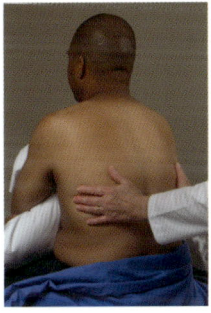
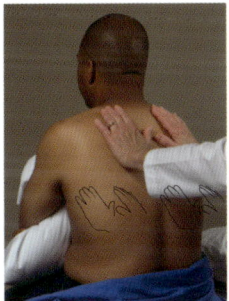

Respiratory excursion.   Tactile fremitus.

Expected Report
- ■ No masses or complaints of pain with palpation of the posterior chest wall
- ■ Respiratory excursion is symmetrical
- ■ Tactile fremitus is felt as a moderate vibration that is stronger between the clavicles as the patient says "99."
  - ■ Note that tactile fremitus is stronger between the clavicles and is expected to decrease as you move your hands downward and outward.

Unexpected Findings: See p. 174.

Percussion
- ■ Use indirect percussion to assess sound tone in the posterior lung fields.
- ■ Use direct or indirect fist percussion to assess for tenderness over each kidney.
  - ■ The kidneys are located in the lower rib cage on each side of the spine in the area known as the costovertebral angle (CVA).
- ■ Percuss for diaphragmatic excursion, using indirect percussion in the following manner:
  1. Ask the patient to take a deep breath and hold it.
  2. Using your non-dominant hand, place the palmar surface of your third finger firmly in the scapular line beneath the right scapula, and slowly move your finger downward as you percuss with your dominant third and fourth fingers while listening for a change in sound from resonance to dullness.

CHEST/ BREASTS

3. Use a felt-tip marker to draw a small mark on the patient's back where the change in sound quality is heard.
4. Ask the patient to "take another deep breath and blow it all the way out and hold it."
5. Begin at the first mark you made, and percuss upward until the sound changes from dull to resonant.
6. Use a felt-tip marker to draw a small mark on the patient's back where the change in sound was heard.
7. Ask the patient to breathe normally a few times.
8. Repeat the process on the left side of the posterior chest.
9. Measure the distance between your upper and lower marks on each side of the posterior chest. *The distance in centimeters between the upper and lower marks represents the extent of diaphragmatic excursion.*

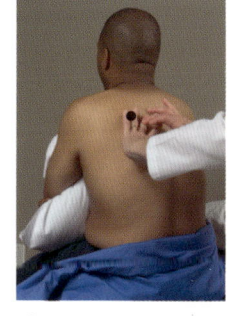

Percuss over posterior lung fields.

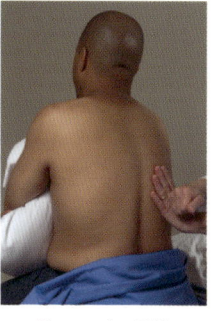

Percuss for CVA tenderness.

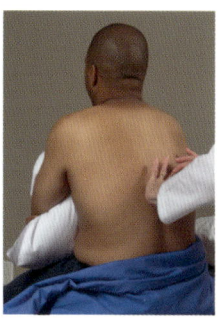

Percuss for diaphragmatic excursion.

Expected Report

- Resonance to percussion is heard over the lung fields of the posterior chest, with a flat note heard over the spinous processes, scapula, and kidneys.
- There is no CVA tenderness.
- Diaphragmatic excursion measures 4 cm bilaterally.

Benign Variations

- Diaphragmatic excursion may measure 3 cm to 6 cm.
  - Note that diaphragmatic excursion may be slightly higher on the right due to the presence of the liver.

Unexpected Findings: See p. 174.

Auscultation

- Ask the patient to look down and cross his arms over his anterior chest or over a small pillow held against his anterior chest to enlarge the posterior chest auscultation area as you:
  1. Auscultate breath sounds over posterior airways and lung fields using the diaphragm of the stethoscope.
  2. Ask the patient to say "99" continuously, as you auscultate symmetrical areas over each lung field.
     - Loud, clear sounds are referred to as "bronchophony" and are abnormal.
  3. Ask the patient to whisper "99" as you auscultate areas over lung fields— evaluate for clarity and symmetry of sounds in right and left lung fields.
     - If sounds are heard clearly, it is referred to as "whispered pectorilo-quy," an abnormal finding.
  4. Ask the patient to say "ee" continuously as you auscultate over the lung fields.
     - If the sound is heard as "ay," it is referred to as "egophony" and is an abnormal finding.

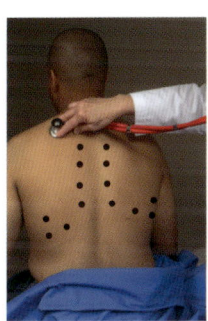

Auscultate posterior lung fields.

Expected Report

- Vesicular breath sounds are heard throughout the lung fields, with medium-pitched bronchovesicular sounds heard over the right main bronchus.
- No bronchophony, whispered pectoriloquy, or egophony is heard.

Unexpected Findings: See p. 174.

Assessing the Breasts

Breast assessment should be performed on males and females.

Inspection

- With the patient seated upright, observe the breasts for:
  - Symmetry
  - Lesions
  - Puckering
  - Size
  - Shape
  - Nipple shape
  - Drainage
- Ask the patent to hold her arms over her head as you observe the breasts for:
  - Symmetry
  - Puckering

Palpation

- With the patient seated upright, use your fingertips to palpate deeply into the axilla, assessing for masses and enlarged lymph nodes. Palpable lymph nodes are assessed for:
  - Size
  - Warmth
  - Mobility
- Place your non-dominant hand under the right breast for support. With the fingertips of your dominant hand, assess for masses and tenderness, using circular motions, beginning at the base of the breast and moving toward the nipple.

- Ask the patient to hold his arms over his head as you palpate the breasts for:
  - Masses
  - Tenderness
- Ask the patient to lie supine with his arms relaxed at his side.
  - **NOTE:** A small pillow or folded towel may be placed under the shoulder on the side of the breast being palpated.
- Use at least one of the techniques shown in the illustrations to palpate each breast for:
  - Masses
  - Tenderness
- Gently squeeze each nipple to check for secretions.

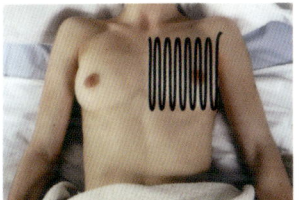 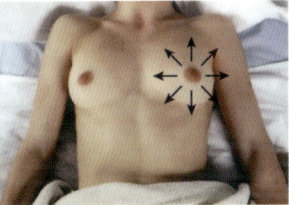

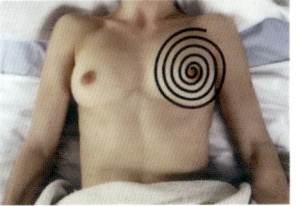

Breast palpation (Dillon, P. (2007). *Nursing health assessment: A critical thinking case studies approach* (2nd ed.). Philadelphia: F.A. Davis Company.)

Expected Report
- Breasts appear symmetrical, medium in size, conical in shape, without lesions or puckering.
- Nipples are everted and without drainage.
- No breast masses are felt.
- There are no palpable masses or lymph nodes in the axilla.
- There is no complaint of breast discomfort during palpation.

Benign Variations
- One breast may be slightly larger than the other.
- In the older adult, changes in breast shape occur due to loss of tissue elasticity.

Unexpected Findings: See pp. 174–175.

Chest and Breasts Assessment Check-Off List

Assessment Task	Performed and Reported Correctly	Performed or Reported Incorrectly	Not Performed
Anterior and Axillary Chest			
Anterior and axillary chest, lesions			
Anterior and axillary chest, scars			
Anterior and axillary chest, deformities			
Chest symmetry			
Anteroposterior (AP) ratio			
Respiratory rate			
Respiratory rhythm or pattern			
Respiratory effort			
Costal angle, measurement			
Anterior and axillary chest, masses			
Anterior and axillary chest, discomfort			

Chest and Breasts Assessment Check-Off List—cont'd

Assessment Task	Performed and Reported Correctly	Performed or Reported Incorrectly	Not Performed
Anterior and axillary chest, crepitus			
Anterior and axillary chest, tactile fremitus			
Anterior respiratory excursion			
Percuss anterior and axillary airways			
Auscultate anterior chest for pitch of sounds over airways and lung fields			
Auscultate anterior chest, inspiratory: expiratory duration comparison in each auscultation area			
Auscultate anterior chest, adventitious sounds: rales, wheezes, rhonchi			
Posterior Chest			
Posterior chest, lesions			
Posterior chest, scars			
Posterior chest, deformities			
Posterior chest, symmetry of movement respiratory movement			
Alignment of the spine			
Description of natural spinal curves			
Posterior chest, masses			
Posterior chest, discomfort to palpation			

Continued

CHEST/
BREASTS

Chest and Breasts Assessment Check-Off List—cont'd

Assessment Task	Performed and Reported Correctly	Performed or Reported Incorrectly	Not Performed
Posterior, respiratory excursion			
Posterior, tactile fremitus			
Posterior chest, percussion sounds			
Posterior chest, CVA tenderness			
Posterior chest, diaphragmatic excursion			
Posterior chest, breath sounds over airways and lung fields			
Posterior chest, bronchophony			
Posterior chest, whispered pectoriloquy			
Posterior chest, egophony			
Breasts			
Breasts, patient seated, symmetry			
Breasts, patient seated, lesions			
Breasts, patient seated, puckering			
Breasts, patient seated, size			
Breasts, patient seated, shape			
Breasts, patient seated, nipple shape			
Breasts, patient seated, drainage			
Breasts, arms held over head, symmetry			

Chest and Breasts Assessment Check-Off List—cont'd

Assessment Task	Performed and Reported Correctly	Performed or Reported Incorrectly	Not Performed
Breasts, arms held over head, puckering			
Axillary lymph nodes, size, warmth, mobility			
Breasts, arms over head, masses			
Breasts, arms held over head, tenderness			
Breasts, patient supine, masses			
Breasts, patient supine, tenderness			
Breasts, nipple, secretions			

Preparing for the Cardiovascular Assessment

Gather Equipment
- Stethoscope
- Felt-tip pen
- Two rulers with mm and cm markings
- Percussion hammer

Prepare Patient
- Explain the procedure.
- Ask the patient to sit upright with his arms at his side for the initial segments of the assessment.
- Clothes should be removed from the upper body, and a drape should be provided.

Examiner
- Stand in front or to the side of the patient.

Assessing Peripheral Circulation

Inspection
- Inspect for edema of the:
  - Face
  - Hands
  - Legs (pretibial)
  - Feet
- Inspect color of:
  - Lips
  - Mucous membranes
  - Nailbeds
- Inspect for capillary refill of nailbeds by pressing the tip of a fingernail or toenail to blanch color and then observing for brisk return of color when the nail is released

Capillary refill.

Expected Report
- There is no edema of the face, hands, legs, or feet.
- Lips, mucous membranes, and nailbeds are pink.
- Nail capillary refill is immediate.

Benign Variations

- Lips may have a blue or brown tint in dark-skinned people.
- Nail capillary refill may be up to 3 seconds.
- Legs and feet may have a slight swelling in older adults after a long day of standing or sitting.

Unexpected Findings: See p. 175.

Assessing the Peripheral Pulses

Peripheral pulse names:

- Temporal
- Carotid—palpate one at a time to avoid occluding brain's arterial blood supply
- Radial
- Brachial
- Femoral
- Popliteal
- Dorsalis pedis
- Posterior tibial

Palpation

- Palpate peripheral pulses, bilaterally and simultaneously, to grade for amplitude or strength.
  - Grading of pulses:
    - **0** Not palpable
    - **1+** Barely palpable
    - **2+** Easily palpable (normal pulse)
    - **3+** Full or increased strength
    - **4+** Bounding
- Palpate a radial pulse to determine:
  - Heart rate
  - Heart rhythm
- Assess for pulse deficit:
  - Have one examiner count the peripheral pulse while a second examiner auscultates the apical pulse.
  - If two examiners are not available, a rough measure of pulse deficit can be determined by a single examiner who counts an apical pulse immediately after counting a peripheral pulse.

CARDIO

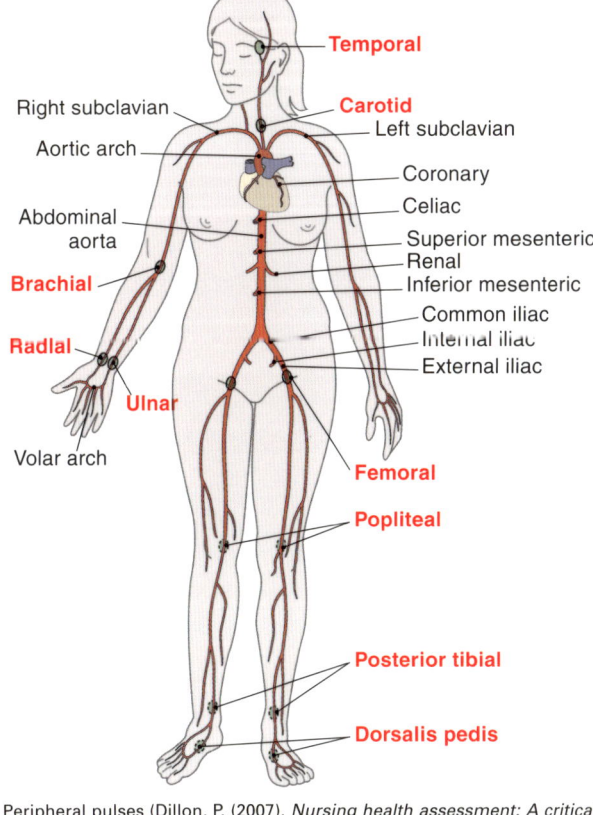

Peripheral pulses (Dillon, P. (2007). *Nursing health assessment: A critical thinking case studies approach* (2nd ed.). Philadelphia: F.A. Davis Company.)

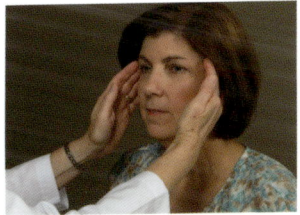

Bilateral palpation of temporal pulses.

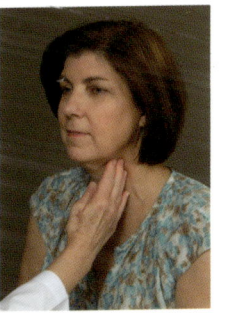

Unilateral palpation of carotid pulse.

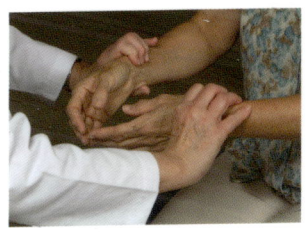

Bilateral palpation of radial pulses.

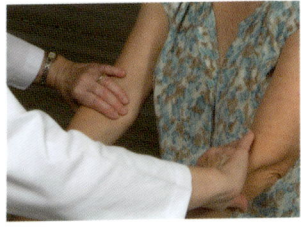

Bilateral palpation of brachial pulses.

CARDIO

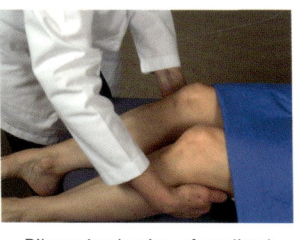

Bilateral palpation of popliteal
pulses.

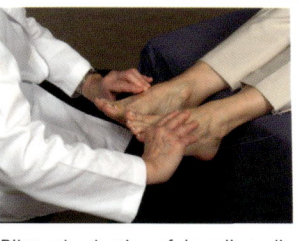

Bilateral palpation of dorsalis pedis
pulses.

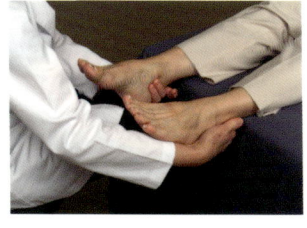

Bilateral palpation of posterior tibial pulses.

Expected Report
- All pulses are 2+ bilaterally.
- The radial pulse rate is 76 and regular in rhythm.
- The radial pulse is equal in rate to the apical pulse.

Benign Variations
- The adult resting pulse rate may range 60 to 100 beats/minute.
- Changes in pulse rate and rhythm vary as the respiratory rate varies.

Unexpected Findings: See p. 176.

Assessing the Temporal Arteries

Auscultation
■ Auscultate the temporal arteries for bruits (pronounced "broo-ees").

Expected Report
■ No temporal bruits heard

Unexpected Findings: See p. 176.

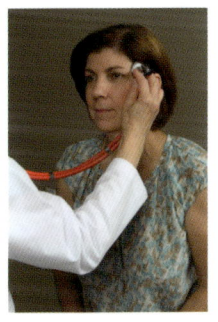

Auscultate for temporal bruits.

Assessing the Carotid Arteries

Auscultation
■ Ask the patient to hold his breath as you auscultate the carotid arteries to assess for bruits.

Expected Report
■ No bruits are detected over the carotid arteries.

Unexpected Findings: See p. 176.

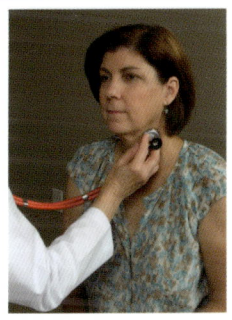

Auscultate for carotid bruits.

CARDIO

Assessing the Precordium

Inspection

- Inspect the precordium (area overlying the heart) to assess for:
  - Lesions
  - Scars
  - Location and size of the apical impulse
    - **NOTE:** Tangential lighting (light that shines across the surface of the skin) is best for inspection of the apical impulse.

Palpation

- Palpate the entire precordium while holding the fingers of the dominant hand together to assess for:
  - The point of maximum impulse (PMI)
    - Usually a penny-sized area in the 5th intercostal space at the left midclavicular line
  - Lifts
  - Heaves
  - Thrills

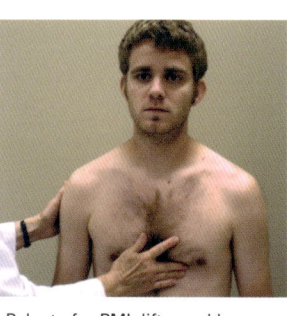

Palpate for PMI, lifts, and heaves.

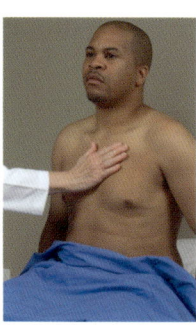

Palpate for thrills.

Expected Report

■ The skin over the chest wall is smooth and without lesions or scars.
■ The apical impulse is approximately 1 cm in diameter and is visible in the left midclavicular line at the 5th intercostal space.
■ The PMI is felt in the 5th intercostal at the left midclavicular line.
■ There are no lifts, heaves, or thrills.

Benign Variations

■ The apical impulse may be in the 4th intercostal space.
■ The apical impulse may be impossible to see or palpate in obese or muscular patients.
■ A thick chest wall may make it difficult to feel the PMI.

Unexpected Findings: See p. 176.

Assessing the Heart Sounds

Cardiac Auscultation: General Guidelines

■ Auscultation should be performed with the diaphragm and the bell of the stethoscope.
■ Auscultation should be performed first with the patient seated and then with the patient supine.
  ■ In this book, instructions for the supine position cardiac auscultation are listed at the end of the cardiac assessment.
■ Auscultation in the left lateral recumbent position intensifies sound by bringing the heart closer to the chest-wall.
■ Sounds are heard best with the aurals (earpieces) of the stethoscope pointed toward the front of the examiner's head.
■ Auscultate the apical heart:
  ■ Rate
  ■ Rhythm
■ Identify S_1 and S_2 (normal sounds that sound like "lup-dup," indicating valve closure) and determine where each is best heard.
  ■ Valve closure is best heard in the direction of blood flow after it passes through the valve, rather than directly over the valve being assessed.
    • S_1 is associated with normal closure of the mitral and tricuspid valves (the atrioventricular [AV] valves) and should be heard best in the mitral area at the apex of the heart (left midclavicular line, 5th intercostal space).

CARDIO

- S_2 is associated with the normal closure of the aortic and pulmonic valves (semilunar valves) and is best heard in the aortic area over the base of the heart (near the upper sternum in the 2nd left intercostal space).
- Auscultate for splitting of S_1 in the tricuspid area (not usually heard in adults)
    - Splitting of S_1 indicates a slight timing difference between closure of the mitral and tricuspid valves
- Auscultate for splitting of S_2 in the pulmonic area
    - Splitting of S_2 indicates a slight timing difference between closure of the aortic and pulmonic valves
- Auscultate for S3 and S4
    - S3 and S4 are known as "gallop" sounds and are best heard with patient in the left lateral decubitus position (supine and positioned on his left side)
        - This position brings the left ventricle nearer to the chest wall.
    - Auscultate for murmurs in the 4 major auscultation areas. They are:
        - Aortic
        - Pulmonic
        - Tricuspid
        - Mitral
        - Murmurs are soft swishing sounds that occur during systole (between S_1 and S_2) or during diastole (between S_2 and S_1) and sound similar to the soft breath sounds that can be auscultated in a healthy infant.
- Auscultate for friction rubs
    - Friction rubs are grating-type sounds.

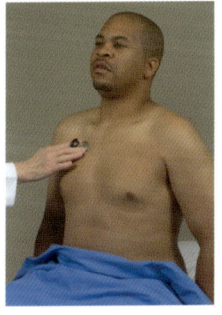

Auscultate aortic valve.

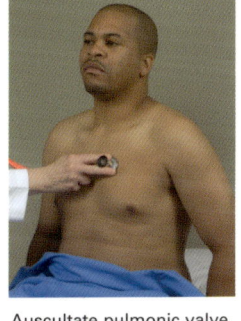

Auscultate pulmonic valve.

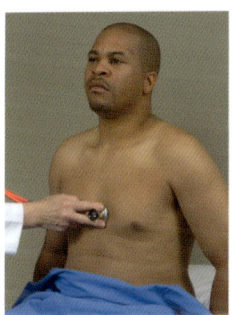

Auscultate tricuspid valve.

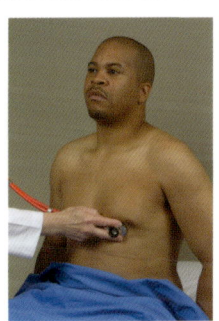

Auscultate mitral valve.

Expected Report

- ■ The heart rate is 68 and is regular in rhythm.
- ■ S_1 and S_2 are heard in all auscultation areas, with S_1 heard best at the apex of the heart and S_2 heard best at the base of the heart.
- ■ No splitting of S_1 or S_2 is heard.
- ■ No murmurs or friction rubs are heard.
- ■ No S_3 or S_4 is heard.

Benign Variations

- S$_3$ may be heard in children, thin young adults, and pregnant women.
- S$_4$ may be heard in athletes.
- Nonpathological S$_3$ and S$_4$ are not generally heard when the patient is sitting upright.

Unexpected Findings: See pp. 176–177.

Assessing the Jugular Veins

Inspection

- Elevate the head of the exam table to about a 45° angle.
- Identify jugular veins
  - Jugular veins empty into the right superior vena cava, then the inferior vena cava, and then into the right atrium of the heart.
  - Steps to identify jugular veins:
    1. Lower the patient's gown or drape to the nipple level to expose the upper sternum.
    2. While standing on the patient's right side, ask the patient to turn his head to the left.
    3. Locate the sternocleidomastoid muscle as the carotid artery and the internal jugular vein run parallel to it and the external jugular vein crosses over it.
    4. Carotid artery pulsations are palpable and have only one observable wave.
    5. Jugular venous pulsations have three visible positive waves (referred to as "undulating") that are easily obliterated with the examiner's fingers.
- Measure jugular venous pressure (JVP)
  - Measurement of the highest level at which the venous pulsation is observed provides an estimation of right heart arterial pressure.
  - JVP may be measured in any position as long as the venous pulsations are visible.
  - Steps to measure jugular venous pressure:
    1. At the angle of Louis, place a ruler perpendicular to the chest. The angle of Louis is at the junction of the manubrium (the most prominent bony landmark on the upper sternum) and the lower sternum near the attachment of the second rib to the sternum.

2. Shine a light across (tangential lighting) the neck vessels to visualize veins.
3. Place a second ruler at the point of the highest level of venous pulsation and allow it to intersect with the first ruler.
4. Measure the distance up from the chest wall to the upper edge of the spot where the two rulers intersect.
   This measurement plus 5 cm estimates central venous pressure. Use a felt-tip pen to mark the measurement.
5. 5 cm is added to the reported measurement because that is the expected distance from the ruler to the middle of the right atrium.

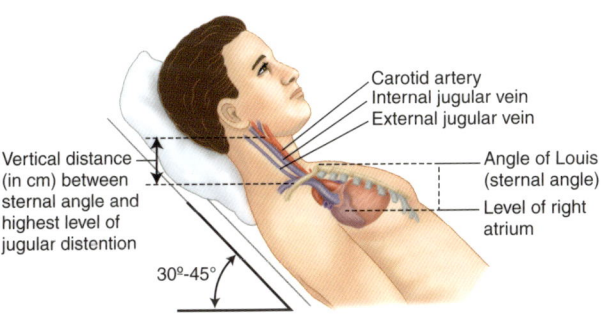

Carotid artery
Internal jugular vein
External jugular vein

Vertical distance (in cm) between sternal angle and highest level of jugular distention

Angle of Louis (sternal angle)
Level of right atrium

30°–45°

Measuring jugular venous pressure (Wilkinson, J. M., & Treas, L. (2011). *Fundamentals of nursing* (2nd ed., Vol. 2, p. 283). F. A. Davis Company.)

Expected Report
■ Jugular venous pressure (JVP) 6 cm

Benign Variations
■ JVP may be up to 8 cm.
■ Note that the JVP is sometimes reported without adding the 5 cm.

Unexpected Findings: See p. 177.

CARDIO

Percussion

■ Place the patient in the left lateral recumbent position to facilitate percussion of the left border of cardiac dullness (LBCD).

■ Begin percussing at the left anterior axillary line and work toward the sternum in the intercostal spaces.

■ Mark the places where the percussion note changes from resonant to dull.

■ The marks indicate the outline of the left border of the heart.

■ Estimation of LBCD is sometimes omitted if the PMI is not displaced lateral to the left midclavicular line.

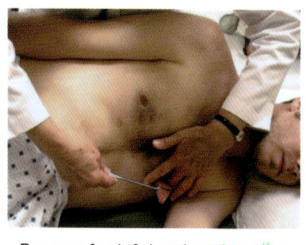

Percuss for left border of cardiac dullness.

Auscultation—Left Lateral Recumbent Position

■ While the patient is in the left lateral recumbent position, auscultate heart for S_3 and S_4.

■ If present, S_3 and S_4 are best heard with the patient in the left lateral recumbent position.

Expected Report

■ Beginning in the left anterior axillary line, the percussion note changes from resonant to dull in the 5th intercostal space at the left midclavicular line.

■ No S_3 or S_4 is detected with the patient in left lateral recumbent position.

Unexpected Findings: See p. 178.

Auscultation—Supine Position

■ Place patient in the supine position
■ Listen for murmurs in the 4 major auscultation areas:

■ Aortic
■ Pulmonic
■ Tricuspid
■ Mitral

- Listen for splitting of S_1 in the mitral area
- Listen for splitting of S_2 in the aortic area
- Auscultate for S_3, S_4
- Listen for friction rubs

Expected Report

- No murmurs are heard.
- There is no splitting of S_1 or S_2.
- No friction rubs are detected.

Unexpected Findings: See p. 178.

Cardiovascular Assessment Check-Off List			
Assessment Task	Performed and Reported Correctly	Performed and Reported Incorrectly	Not Performed
Peripheral Circulation			
Edema, face			
Edema, hands			
Edema, legs			
Edema, feet			
Color, lips and mucous membranes			
Color, nailbeds			
Peripheral Pulses			
Capillary refill, nailbed			
Temporal pulses, palpate bilateral & grade			
Carotid pulses, palpate unilateral & grade			
Radial pulses, palpate & grade			
Brachial pulses, palpate bilateral & grade			

Continued

CARDIO

Cardiovascular Assessment Check-Off List—cont'd

Assessment Task	Performed and Reported Correctly	Performed and Reported Incorrectly	Not Performed
Femoral pulses, palpate bilateral & grade			
Popliteal pulses, palpate bilateral & grade			
Posterior tibial pulses, palpate bilateral & grade			
Dorsalis pedis pulses, palpate bilateral & grade			
Radial pulse rate, palpate & grade			
Radial pulse rhythm, palpate & grade			
Temporal & Carotid Arteries			
Radial/apical pulse deficit, palpate and auscultate			
Temporal bruits, auscultate			
Carotid bruits, auscultate			
Precordium			
Precordium, inspect for lesions			
Precordium, inspect for scars			
Apical impulse, inspect for location and size			
Precordium, palpate for PMI			
Precordium, palpate for lifts			
Precordium, palpate for heaves			
Precordium, palpate for thrills			

Cardiovascular Assessment Check-Off List—cont'd

Assessment Task	Performed and Reported Correctly	Performed and Reported Incorrectly	Not Performed
Heart Sounds			
Auscultate, heart rate			
Auscultate, heart rhythm			
S_1 and S_2, auscultate for loudest location			
S_1 and S_2, auscultate for splitting			
S_3 and S_4, auscultate for			
Aortic valve, auscultate for			
Pulmonic valve, auscultate for murmur			
Tricuspid valve, auscultate for murmur			
Mitral valve, auscultate for murmur			
Friction rub, auscultate for			
Jugular Veins (patient at 45°)			
Jugular venous pressure, measure JVP			
Jugular Veins (patient left lateral recumbent)			
LBCD, percuss for			
S_3 and S_4, auscultate for			
Jugular Veins (patient supine)			
Inspect for lifts and heaves			
Aortic valve, auscultate using stethoscope diaphragm			

Continued

CARDIO

Cardiovascular Assessment Check-Off List—cont'd

Assessment Task	Performed and Reported Correctly	Performed and Reported Incorrectly	Not Performed
Pulmonic valve, auscultate using stethoscope diaphragm			
Tricuspid valve, auscultate using stethoscope diaphragm			
Mitral valve, auscultate using stethoscope diaphragm			
S_1 and S_2, auscultate for splitting in mitral area			
S_2 auscultate for splitting in the aortic area			
S_3 and S_4, auscultate for			
Friction rubs, auscultate for			

Preparing for the Abdomen Assessment

Gather Equipment
- Penlight
- Stethoscope
- Small ruler with mm and cm markings
- Felt-tipped pen
- Percussion hammer

Prepare Patient
- Explain the procedure.
- Place the patient in the supine position with his arms at his side.
- Expose the abdomen and place a drape over the patient's chest and below the anterior edge of the symphysis pubis.
- Ask the patient to bend his knees and place his feet flat on the end of the exam table to help the abdomen relax.

Examiner
- Stand at the patient's right side. The left-handed examiner should stand at the patient's left side.

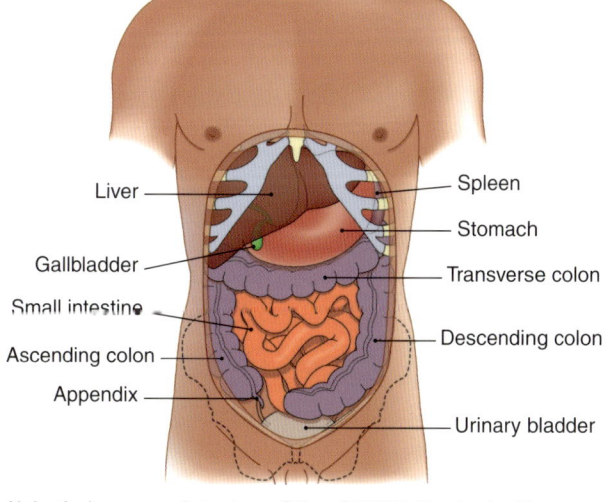

Liver

Gallbladder

Small intestine

Ascending colon

Appendix

Spleen

Stomach

Transverse colon

Descending colon

Urinary bladder

Abdominal organs and structures (Dillon, P. (2007). *Nursing health assessment: A critical thinking case studies approach* (2 ed.). Philadelphia: F. A. Davis Company.)

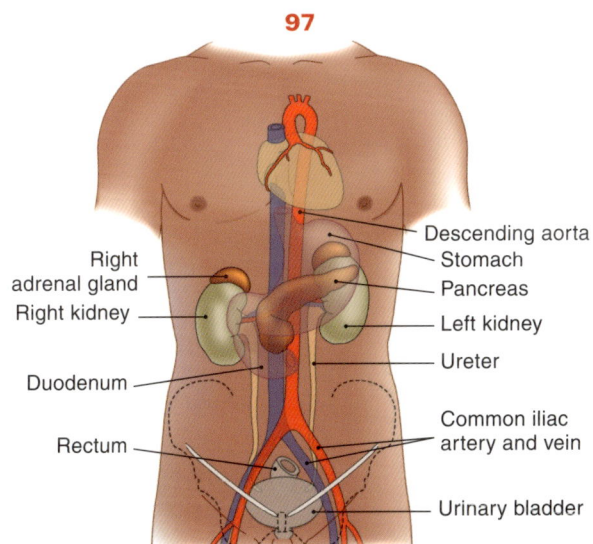

Right adrenal gland

Right kidney

Duodenum

Rectum

Descending aorta

Stomach

Pancreas

Left kidney

Ureter

Common iliac artery and vein

Urinary bladder

Other abdominal organs and structures (Dillon, P. (2007). *Nursing health assessment: A critical thinking case studies approach* (2 ed.). Philadelphia: F. A. Davis Company.)

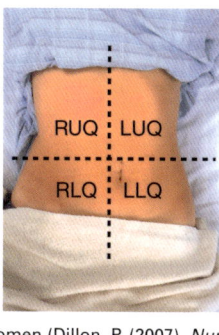

Four quadrants of abdomen (Dillon, P. (2007). *Nursing health assessment: A critical thinking case studies approach* (2 ed.). Philadelphia: F. A. Davis Company.)

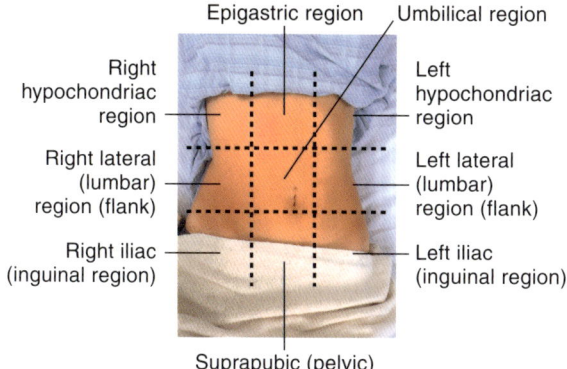

Epigastric region   Umbilical region

Right hypochondriac region   Left hypochondriac region

Right lateral (lumbar) region (flank)   Left lateral (lumbar) region (flank)

Right iliac (inguinal region)   Left iliac (inguinal region)

Suprapubic (pelvic) (hypogastric) region

Nine regions of abdomen (Dillon, P. (2007). *Nursing health assessment: A critical thinking case studies approach* (2 ed.). Philadelphia: F. A. Davis Company.).

Assessing the Abdomen

Inspection

- Inspect abdomen for:
  - Symmetry
  - Skin color
  - Scars
  - Lesions
  - Abdominal contour
  - Umbilicus
- With the patient supine, shine a penlight across the abdomen as you view abdomen tangentially (lower your head so that you are looking "across" the patient's abdomen) to check for:
  - Peristalsis
  - Pulsations
  - Bulging
  - Visible masses
  - Enlarged veins

Expected Report

- The abdomen is symmetrical and slightly rounded with no visible scars, lesions, bulges, visible masses, or enlarged veins.
- The umbilicus is midline and inverted.
- There is no visible abdominal peristalsis or pulsation.

Benign Variations

- In thin patients, the abdomen may appear flat or slightly sunken.
- A slightly everted umbilicus is considered normal.
- Slight movements of peristalsis and slight aortic pulsation may be visible in thin patients.

Unexpected Findings: See pp. 178–179.

Auscultation—Using Stethoscope's Bell

Note: Unlike assessment of other areas, auscultation of the abdomen is performed BEFORE percussion and palpation to avoid stimulation of peristalsis and to avoid the possibility of eliciting pain at the beginning of the assessment.

- Auscultate for aortic bruits.
  - Located in the epigastric area
  - Bruits are swishing sounds similar to that of cardiac murmur

ABDOMEN

- Auscultate the renal arteries for bruits bilaterally.
  - Located just below the 12th or lowest rib, lateral to the epigastric area in the right and left upper abdominal quadrants
- Auscultate the iliac arteries for bruits.
  - Located lateral and inferior to the umbilicus in the right and left lower quadrants
- Auscultate the femoral arteries for bruits.
  - Located in right and left groin, slightly medial to nipple line on each side
- Auscultate for peritoneal friction rubs.
  - Located over the liver, spleen, and, if present, masses
  - Friction rubs are grating sounds indicating inflammation, infection, or abnormal growths

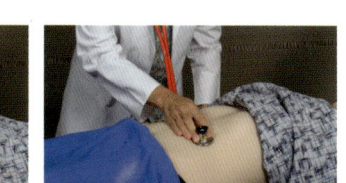

Auscultate for aortic bruits.

Auscultate for renal bruits.

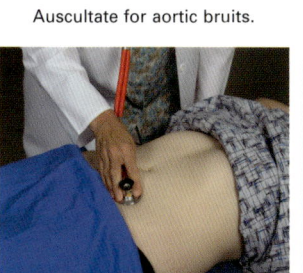

Auscultate for iliac bruits.

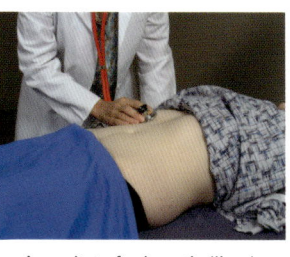

Auscultate for hepatic (liver) friction rub.

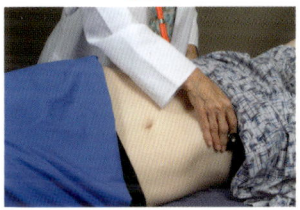

Auscultate for splenic friction rubs.

Expected Report
- No aortic, renal, iliac, or femoral bruits are heard.
- No liver or splenic friction rubs are heard.

Unexpected Findings: See p. 179.

Auscultation—Using Stethoscope's Diaphragm
- Auscultate for bowel sounds in all four quadrants.
  - Listen for at least a full minute before reporting that bowel sounds are not heard in any quadrant.
  - **NOTE:** Bowel sounds caused by peristalsis in one quadrant may result in sounds being transmitted to other quadrants, especially in patients with little abdominal fat.

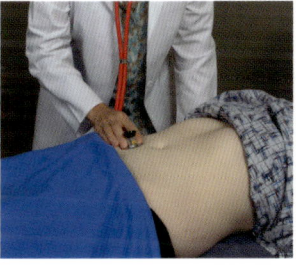

Auscultate for bowel sounds in all 4 quadrants.

Expected Report
- Bowel sounds, 6 to 10 low-pitched clicks and gurgles per minute, are heard in all 4 abdominal quadrants.

Benign Variations
- Frequency of bowel sounds may normally be 3 to 35/minute.

Unexpected Findings: See p. 179.

ABDOMEN

Percussion (Indirect)

NOTE: Painful areas are percussed last. All areas are percussed for tone.

- Percuss all 4 abdominal quadrants; 3 to 4 places in each quadrant, including lateral and medial areas.
- Percuss to estimate size of the liver.
  - Beginning under the right nipple, percuss downward along the midclavicular line (MCL) until the percussion sound quality changes from resonance to dullness. The dull sound denotes the upper border of the liver.
  - Use a felt-tipped pen to place a mark at the point where the sound changes from resonance to a dull quality.
  - Beginning to the right and lateral to the umbilicus, percuss upward along the MCL until tympany changes to dullness. The dull sound denotes the lower border of the liver.
  - Place a mark at the point where the sound changes to a dull quality. The total area of dullness represents the liver span.
  - If assessment of liver descent is desired, ask the patient to take a deep breath and hold it while you percuss upward from the umbilical level at the midclavicular line to approximate the location of the lower border of the liver.
- Percuss to estimate the size of the spleen.
  - Beginning just posterior to the left midaxillary line at the 3rd intercostal space, percuss downward until tympany or resonance changes to dullness and then changes back to tympany.
    - Place a mark at each point where the sound quality changes. The area of dullness represents the span of the spleen.
- Percuss to assess for bladder distention.
  - Beginning at the symphysis pubis, percuss upward to the umbilicus, noting any dullness. Dullness represents the space occupied by urine in the bladder.

Percuss the abdomen in all 4 quadrants.

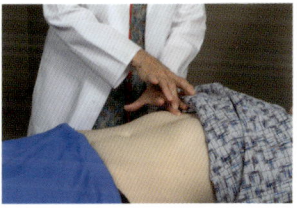

Percuss downward to locate upper liver border.

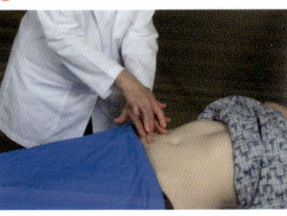

Percuss upward to locate lower liver border.

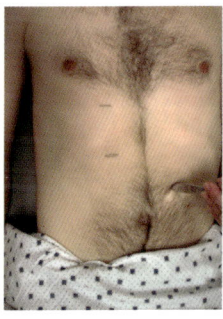

Estimation of liver size.

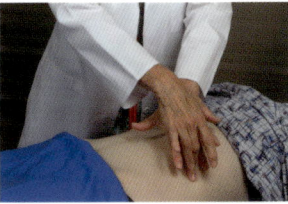

Percuss to estimate spleen size.

Expected Report
- Tympany predominates in all 4 abdominal quadrants.
- Dullness to percussion is heard in the right midclavicular line (R MCL) beginning at the 6th intercostal space and continuing to approximately 2 cm below the right costal margin.
- Estimated liver span at R MCL is 8 cm.
- Dullness to percussion is heard near the left midaxillary line between the 6th and 10th ribs.

ABDOMEN

Benign Variations

■ Liver span may be 6 to 12 centimeters.
■ Dullness in unexpected areas of the abdomen may be caused by fecal material in the colon.
■ Percussion near the left midaxillary line is unreliable for estimation of spleen size because a full or empty stomach or colon may mimic or obscure splenic percussion dullness.

Unexpected Findings: See p. 179.

Palpation

■ Techniques to help the patient relax for abdominal palpation include:
  ■ Asking the patient to bend his knees and place his feet flat on the exam table
  ■ Asking the patient to place his own hand on his abdomen and placing your hand on top of his to demonstrate how palpation will feel
  ■ Asking the patient to take several slow deep breaths so that you can palpate during expiration
■ Lightly palpate all 4 quadrants, pressing down 1 to 2 cm, noting any:
  ■ Tenderness
  ■ Superficial masses
    • Size
    • Consistency
    • Mobility
  ■ Crepitus
■ Deeply palpate all 4 quadrants, pressing down 4 to 6 cm, noting any:
  ■ Tenderness
  ■ Masses
    • Size
    • Consistency
    • Mobility
  ■ Beginning at the level of the umbilicus, in the R MCL, palpate upward toward the R costal margin with your fingertips held together until detecting the firmness of the lower border of the liver.
  ■ Beginning at the level of the umbilicus, just lateral to the L MCL, palpate upward toward the L costal margin to check for splenic enlargement.
  ■ Also attempt to capture the lower border of the spleen between the fingers of your right and left hands as shown in the illustration.
  ■ Note that the spleen should be non-palpable.
■ Note the location, size, consistency, and mobility of any masses.

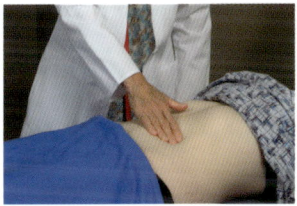

Lightly palpate all 4 abdominal quadrants.

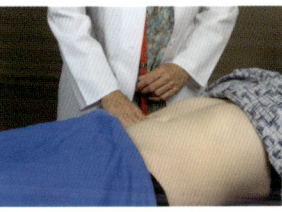

Deeply palpate all 4 abdominal quadrants.

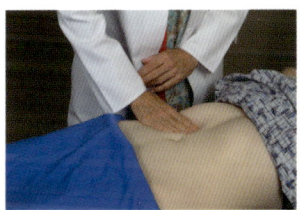

Palpate upward for the lower liver border.

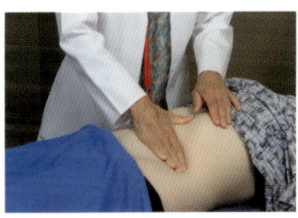

Palpate upward for splenic enlargement.

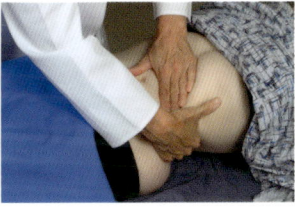

Attempt to capture the spleen.

ABDOMEN

Expected Report

- No abdominal masses are detected by light or deep palpation.
  - The lower edge of the liver is palpable 2 cm below the right MCL.
  - The spleen is non-palpable.

Benign Variations

- The lower edge of the liver may not be palpable or may be less than 2 cm below the right MCL.
- The tip of the spleen may be palpable below the left midaxillary costal margin.

Unexpected Findings: See p. 179.

Scratch Test — Abdomen

- The scratch test is an alternate method for estimating the size of solid organs or masses and is most useful when assessing a thin patient.
- The scratch test is performed by using landmarks described in the directions for abdominal percussion and palpation.
- Place your stethoscope below or outside potential or expected organ borders, and use one finger to make a light scratching motion on the abdominal wall beside the stethoscope, slowly moving the stethoscope and your finger along the same path followed during percussion.
  - The sound heard will be magnified when moving away from a solid organ to an air-filled area.

Scratch test.

Superficial Abdominal Reflexes

- The abdominal reflexes tests are neurological tests.
- Assess abdominal reflexes in each abdominal quadrant by beginning near the umbilicus and stroking away from the umbilicus, upward or downward in the same quadrant, with the end of a percussion hammer or tongue blade.

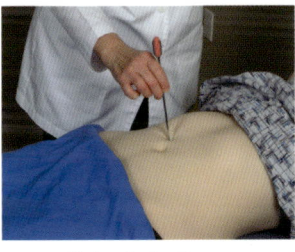

Abdominal reflexes.

Expected Report

- The umbilicus moves slightly toward each area of stimulation in each quadrant with assessment of superficial abdominal reflexes.

Benign Variations

- Superficial abdominal reflexes may be diminished in obese patients or patients whose abdomens have been stretched during pregnancy.
- These reflexes may be difficult or impossible to elicit.

Unexpected Findings: See p. 180.

Inguinal Lymph Nodes

Palpation

- Assess for inguinal lymph nodes by holding your fingers together and using moderate pressure to palpate the inguinal areas, horizontally and vertically along the upper anterior and medial edges of each thigh.

ABDOMEN

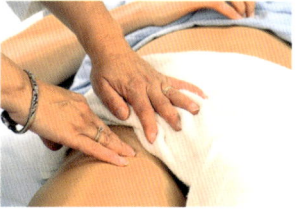

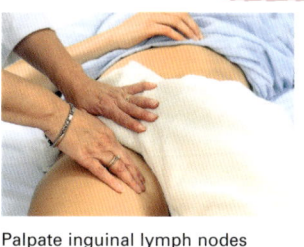

Palpate inguinal lymph nodes (Dillon, P. (2007). *Nursing health assessment: A critical thinking case studies approach* (2nd ed.). Philadelphia: F. A. Davis Company.)

Palpate inguinal lymph nodes (Dillon, P. (2007). *Nursing health assessment: A critical thinking case studies approach* (2nd ed.). Philadelphia: F. A. Davis Company.)

Expected Report
■ No tenderness or palpable nodes noted in the inguinal areas

Benign Variations
■ Shotty (1 to 2 cm, hard, mobile) nodes

Unexpected Findings: See p. 180.

Abdomen Assessment Check-Off List			
Assessment Task	**Performed and Reported Correctly**	**Performed or Reported Incorrectly**	**Not Performed**
Inspection			
Abd skin, color			
Abd skin, scars,			
Abd skin, lesions			
Contour			
Umbilicus			
Peristalsis			
Pulsations			
Bulging			

Abdomen Assessment Check-Off List—cont'd

Assessment Task	Performed and Reported Correctly	Performed or Reported Incorrectly	Not Performed
Masses			
Veins			
Auscultation			
Auscultate, aortic bruits			
Auscultate renal bruits			
Auscultate iliac artery bruits			
Auscultate femoral artery bruits			
Auscultate peritoneal friction rub			
Auscultate, bowel sounds, 4 quadrants			
Percussion			
Percuss, 4 quadrants			
Percuss, lower border, liver			
Percuss, spleen size			
Percuss, bladder			
Palpation			
Palpate, lightly, 4 quadrants			
Palpate, deeply, 4 quadrants			
Palpate, liver			
Palpate, spleen			
Scratch test			
Superficial abdominal reflexes			
Inguinal lymph nodes, palpate for size and tenderness			

ABDOMEN

Preparing for the Musculoskeletal Assessment

Gather Equipment

- Goniometer may be used to measure range of motion

Prepare Patient

- Explain procedure
- Patient is standing, seated, or supine as appropriate during various parts of the assessment.
- Positions shown in this publication are optional (may be performed with the patient in a position different from the one shown) for some parts of the musculoskeletal physical assessment.

Examiner

- Stand in front of, behind, or to the side of the patient as needed to assess the musculoskeletal system

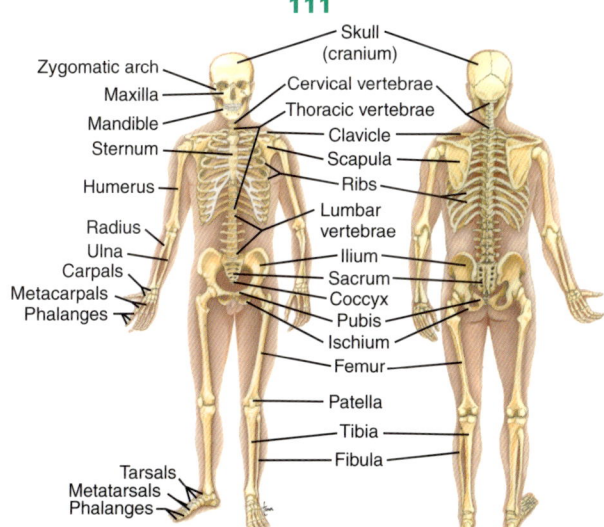

Skull
(cranium)

Zygomatic arch

Maxilla

Mandible

Sternum

Humerus

Radius

Ulna

Carpals

Metacarpals

Phalanges

Cervical vertebrae

Thoracic vertebrae

Clavicle

Scapula

Ribs

Lumbar
vertebrae

Ilium

Sacrum

Coccyx

Pubis

Ischium

Femur

Patella

Tibia

Fibula

Tarsals

Metatarsals

Phalanges

Skeleton. Anterior view. Posterior view (Scanlon, V. C., & Sanders, T. (2010). *Essentials of anatomy and physiology* (Sixth ed.). Philadelphia: F. A. Davis Company.)

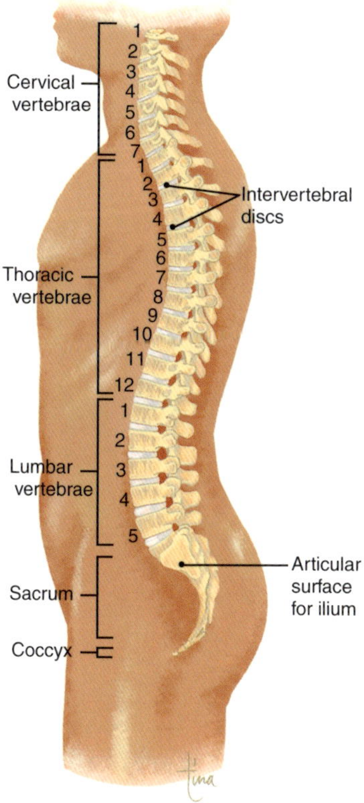

Cervical
vertebrae

1
2
3
4
5
6
7

Intervertebral
discs

1
2
3
4
5
6
7
8
9
10
11
12

Thoracic
vertebrae

Lumbar
vertebrae

1
2
3
4
5

Sacrum

Articular
surface
for ilium

Coccyx

Vertebral column (Scanlon, V. C., & Sanders, T. (2010). *Essentials of
anatomy and physiology* (Sixth ed.). Philadelphia: F. A. Davis Company.)

112

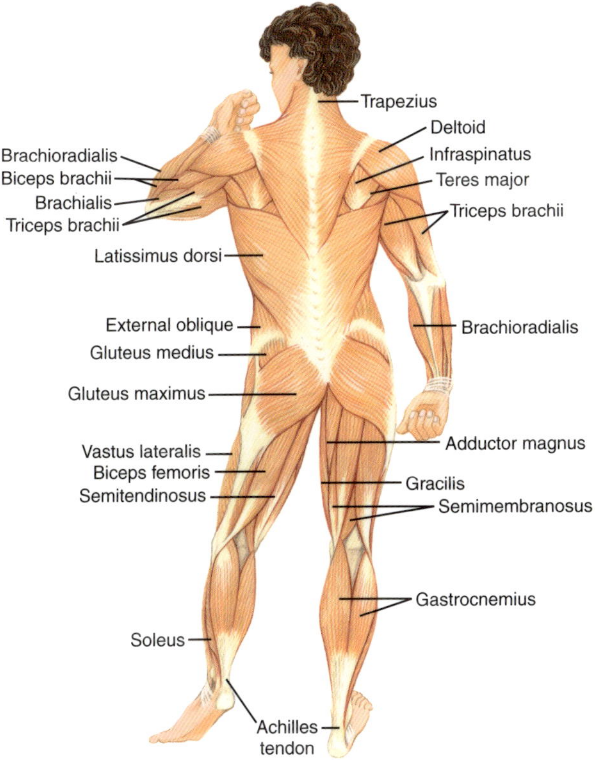

Trapezius

Deltoid

Infraspinatus

Teres major

Brachioradialis

Biceps brachii

Brachialis

Triceps brachii

Triceps brachii

Latissimus dorsi

External oblique

Brachioradialis

Gluteus medius

Gluteus maximus

Vastus lateralis

Adductor magnus

Biceps femoris

Gracilis

Semitendinosus

Semimembranosus

Gastrocnemius

Soleus

Achilles
tendon

Major muscles of the body: posterior view (Scanlon, V. C., & Sanders, T.
(2010). *Essentials of anatomy and physiology* (Sixth ed.). Philadelphia:
F. A. Davis Company.)

MUSCULO-
SKELETAL

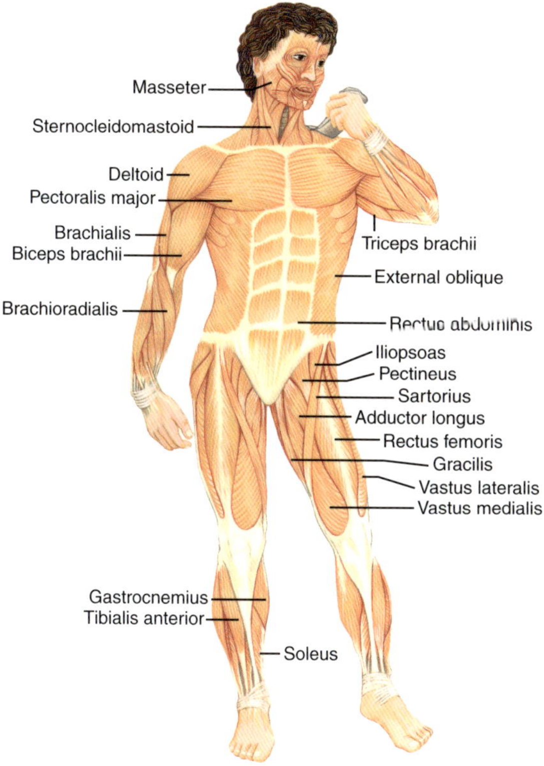

Masseter

Sternocleidomastoid

Deltoid

Pectoralis major

Brachialis

Biceps brachii

Brachioradialis

Triceps brachii

External oblique

Rectus abdominis

Iliopsoas

Pectineus

Sartorius

Adductor longus

Rectus femoris

Gracilis

Vastus lateralis

Vastus medialis

Gastrocnemius

Tibialis anterior

Soleus

Major muscles of the body: anterior view (Scanlon, V. C., & Sanders, T. (2010). *Essentials of anatomy and physiology* (Sixth ed.). Philadelphia: F. A. Davis Company.)

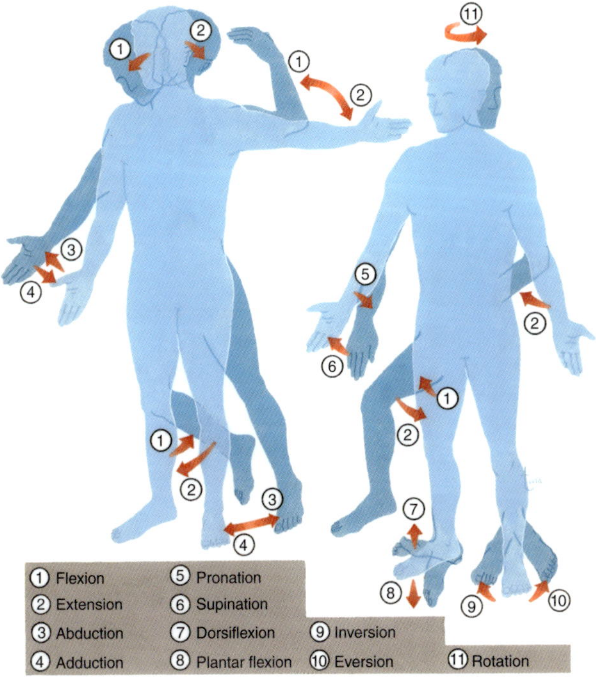

Actions of muscles (Scanlon, V. C., & Sanders, T. (2010). *Essentials of anatomy and physiology* (Sixth ed.) Philadelphia: F. A. Davis Company.)

1 Flexion	5 Pronation	
2 Extension	6 Supination	
3 Abduction	7 Dorsiflexion	9 Inversion
4 Adduction	8 Plantar flexion	10 Eversion
		11 Rotation

MUSCULO-SKELETAL

Assessing the Musculoskeletal System

Assessing Symmetry, Posture, Alignment, and Equilibrium

Inspection

- Ask patient to stand
- Compare each side of the body and extremities to the opposite side for:
  - Gross symmetry
  - Posture
- Observe:
  - Head alignment with shoulders
  - Spinal alignment and curves
  - Equilibrium
    - To assess equilibrium, perform the Romberg test: Ask the patient to stand with his eyes closed, feet together, and arms at his sides.
      - For maximum safety, the patient may be asked to stand facing an exam table or near a wall.
    - For 20 seconds, stand by the patient with your arms encircling but not touching him or her to catch the patient if balance is lost. If the patient loses balance during the Romberg test, gait and tandem heel-to-toe walking should not be tested.

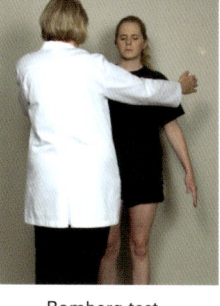

Romberg test.

Expected Report

- Body is grossly symmetrical
- Posture is erect with shoulders held back and knees slightly bent
- Head is in alignment with shoulders
- Spine is midline
- Cervical spine is slightly concave, thoracic spine is slightly convex, and lumbar spine is slightly concave
- Swaying is minimal as the patient stands with his eyes closed
- Romberg test negative

Benign Variations
- Slight gross asymmetry of the body is common.

Unexpected Findings: See p. 180.

Assessing Gait

Inspection
- Observe usual gait.
  - Ask the patient to walk several steps as you observe gait; this is an assessment of both musculoskeletal and neurological function.
- Observe tandem heel-to-toe walking.
  - Ask the patient to walk several steps using heel-to-toe steps.
  - This is an assessment of both musculoskeletal and neurological function.

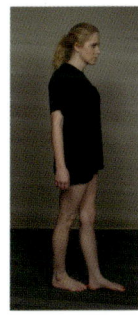

Tandem heel to toe walk.

- Observe tiptoe walking.
  - Ask the patient to walk on tiptoes.

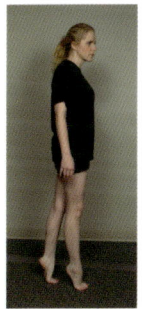

Tip toe walk.

MUSCULO-SKELETAL

- Observe balancing on heels
  - Ask the patient to balance on his heels.

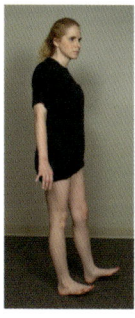

Balance on heels.

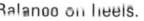

Expected Report
- Gait is steady with toes pointing forward.
- Tandem heel-to-toe walk is accurate with no loss of balance.
- Patient walks on tiptoes and balances on heels.

Benign Variations
- Toes may point slightly inward or outward as the patient walks.
- Tandem heel-to-toe walk may cause some loss of balance in the older adult, so care should be taken to prevent falls.

Unexpected Findings: See p. 180.

Assessing Upper and Lower Extremity Muscle Strength

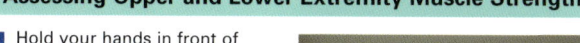

- Hold your hands in front of the patient, with your fingers pointing toward the patient.
- Ask patient to grip the fingers of both your hands as firmly as possible.
  - Note strength and symmetry of grip.

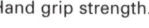

Hand grip strength.

118

- Hold your hands in front of the patient, with your palms facing each other and about 8 inches apart.
- Ask the patient to push your hands together.
  - Note symmetry and strength of the medial pushing movement.

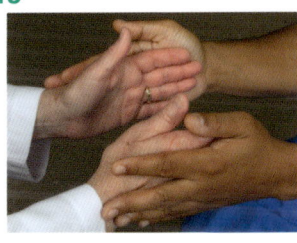

Upper extremity push hands together.

- Ask the patient to push your hands farther apart.
  - Note symmetry and strength of the lateral pushing movement.

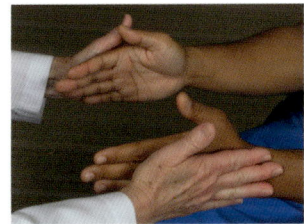

Upper extremity push hands apart.

- Flex your elbows 90°, holding your hands about the level of your shoulders.
- Ask the patient to pull your hands or lower arms toward himself.
- Note symmetry and strength of the pulling motion.

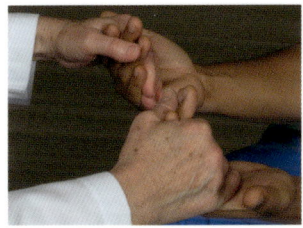

Upper extremity pull.

MUSCULO-SKELETAL

- Ask the patient to push your hands toward yourself.
  - Note symmetry and strength of the pushing motion.

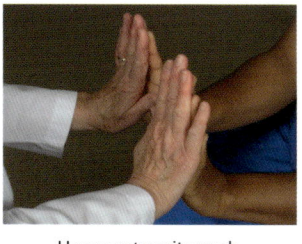

Upper extremity push.

- Place your hands behind the patient's lower legs.
- Ask the patient to pull his lower legs backward.
  - Note symmetry and strength of the pulling movement.

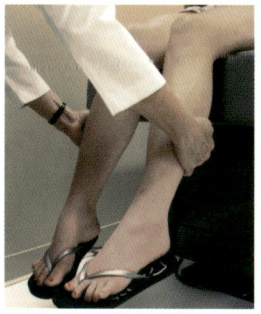

Lower extremity strength pull.

- Place your hands against the front of the patient's lower legs.
- Ask the patient to push his lower legs forward.
  - Note symmetry and strength of the pushing movement.

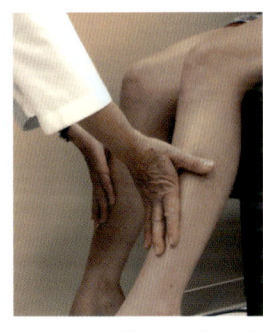

Lower extremity strength push.

Expected Report
- Pushing and pulling movements strong and symmetrical in all extremities

Unexpected Findings: See p. 180.

Assessing Mobile Joints

Inspection and Palpation
- Beginning at the head and moving toward the toes, perform a gross inspection of all joints for:
  - Redness
  - Deformity
- Gently palpate all joints for:
  - Excess warmth
  - Tenderness

Expected Report (for each joint)
- There is no redness or deformity of the joints.
- There is no excess warmth of the joints.
- There is no tenderness of the joints.

Unexpected Findings for All Mobile Joints: See pp. 180–181.

MUSCULO-SKELETAL

Mobile Joints—Range of Motion

In the remainder of the musculoskeletal assessment, beginning at the head and moving to the toes, instruct the patient how to move each joint through its entire range of motion (ROM). As the patient moves through the motions:

■ Observe for symmetry in the complete joint ROM.
■ Listen for crepitus.

NOTE: ROM may be performed passively (examiner moves the joints) or actively (patient moves the joints) or both. Patients who are experiencing pain or weakness may have limited active movement of the musculoskeletal system.

Expected Report
■ Expected ROM of mobile joints is noted in the sections below.

Benign Variations
■ Crepitus of a joint may be associated with advanced age, when joint cartilage becomes thin and joint lubricating fluids are decreased.

Unexpected Findings: See pp. 180–181.

Assessing the Temporomandibular Joint (Jaw)

Inspection
Ask patient to:

■ Move his lower jaw forward (jaw protraction).

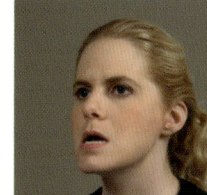

Temporomandibular joint (TMJ or jaw) protraction.

■ Move his lower jaw toward the spine (jaw retraction).

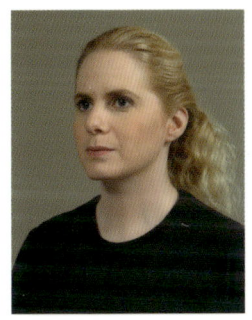

TMJ or jaw retraction.

■ Open his mouth (jaw extension).

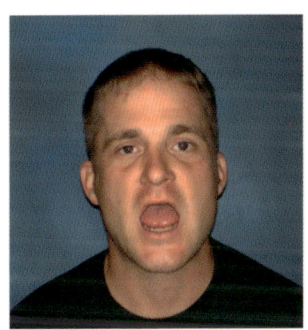

TMJ or jaw extension.

MUSCULO-SKELETAL

- Move his lower jaw side to side (jaw lateral excursion).

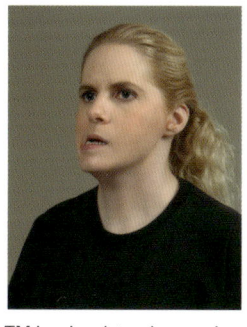

TMJ or jaw lateral excursion.

Expected Report
- Projects, retracts, extends, and moves lower jaw side to side with ease and without crepitus

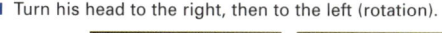

Assessing the Cervical Spine (Neck)

Inspection
Ask patient to:

- Turn his head to the right, then to the left (rotation).

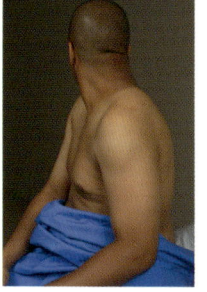

Neck rotation.

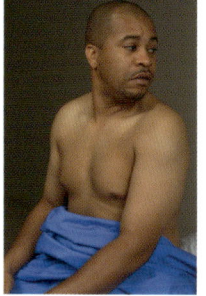

Neck rotation.

■ Flex his head forward by moving the chin close to the chest (forward flexion).

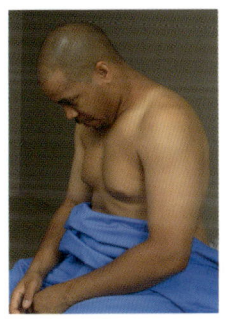

Neck forward flexion.

■ Extend the head backward by moving the chin away from the chest (extension).

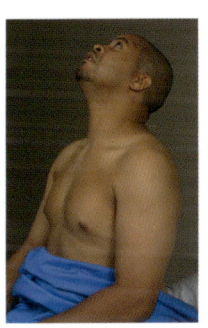

Neck extension.

MUSCULO-SKELETAL

■ Move his right ear toward right shoulder without moving shoulder, and then move left ear as far as possible toward left shoulder (lateral flexion).

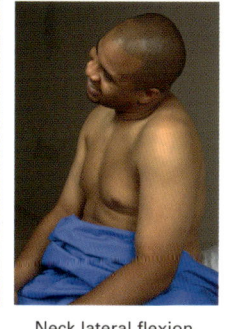

Neck lateral flexion. Neck lateral flexion.

Expected Report
■ Moves neck through rotation, forward and lateral flexion, and extension with ease and without crepitus

Assessing the Shoulders

Inspection
Ask patient to:

■ Hold his arms out straight in front of his body (shoulder flexion).

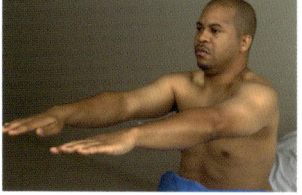

Shoulder flexion.

- Hold his arms straight and behind his body (shoulder extension).

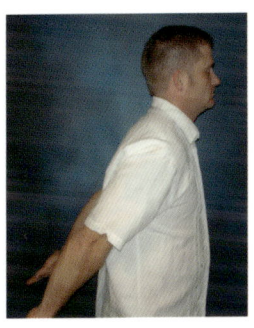

Shoulder extension.

- Extend his elbows to straighten his arms outward, at 90° to the body, then lift his arms upward to place hands together over his head (shoulder abduction).

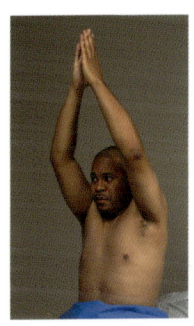

Shoulder abduction.

MUSCULO-SKELETAL

- Move both arms across the front of the body so that hands rest in the opposite axilla or on the opposite shoulder (shoulder adduction).

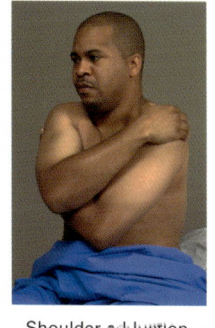

Shoulder adduction.

- Extend his elbows to straighten arms outward, at 90° to the body, and then draw wide imaginary circles (shoulder circumduction).

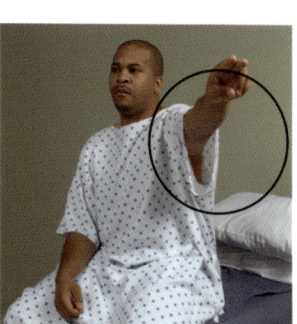

Shoulder circumduction.

- Hold his upper arms against his sides, and then flex the elbow 90° as he extends his hands and forearms outward. You may gently push his hands outward if he is unable to do this. Note that the upper arms remain against the body (shoulder external rotation).

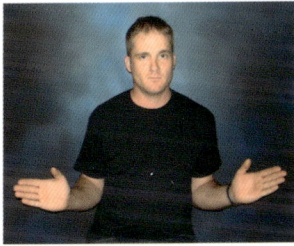

Shoulder external shoulder rotation.

- Place his thumbs on his lower spine, and move his thumbs upward on the spine as far as possible (shoulder internal rotation).

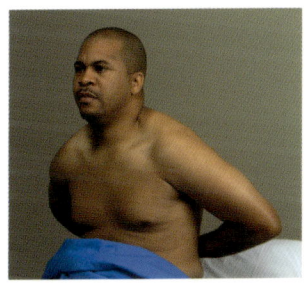

Shoulder internal shoulder rotation.

Expected Report
- Moves shoulders symmetrically through flexion, extension, abduction, adduction, circumduction, external rotation, and internal rotation, with ease and without crepitus

MUSCULO-SKELETAL

Assessing the Elbows

Inspection
Ask patient to:

- Hold his arms straight (elbow extension).

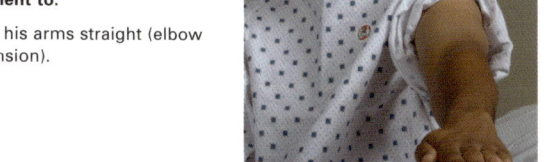

Elbow extension.

- Turn the palms of his hands upward (elbow supination).

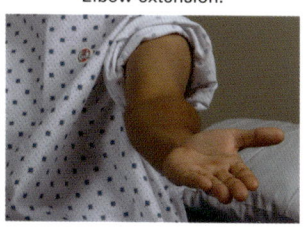

Elbow supination.

- Turn the palms of his hands downward (elbow pronation).

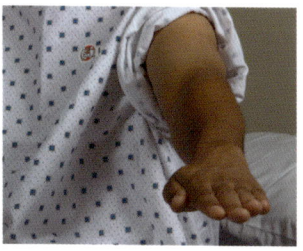

Elbow pronation.

- Move his hands to touch each ipsilateral (same side) shoulder (elbow flexion).

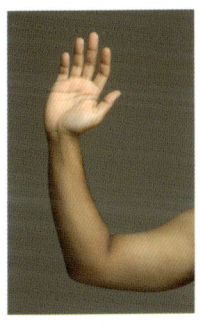

Elbow flexion.

Expected Report
- Moves elbows symmetrically through extension, supination, pronation, and flexion with ease and without crepitus

Assessing the Wrists

Inspection
Ask patient to stand or sit with arms extended in front of his body and:

- Turn the palms of his hands so that the palms of his hands face upward (wrist supination).

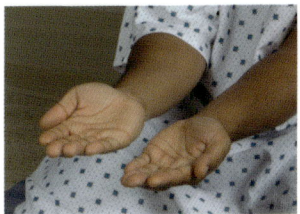

Wrist supination.

■ Rotate his wrists so that his palms face downward (wrist pronation).

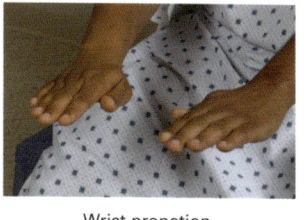

Wrist pronation.

■ Holding his elbows extended in front of his torso at a 180°-angle, move his hands and fingers to point toward the floor (wrist flexion).

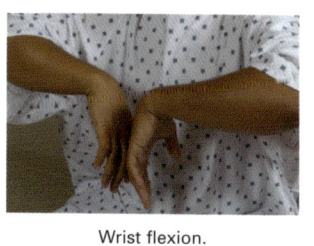

Wrist flexion.

■ Holding his elbows extended in front of his torso at a 180°-angle, move his hands and fingers to point upward (wrist extension).

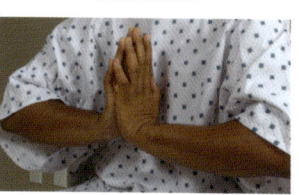

Wrist extension.

- Holding his arms in front of the torso, move his hands and fingers medially (inward) without moving his arms (wrist radial deviation).

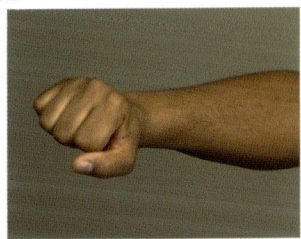

Wrist radial deviation.

- Holding his arms in front of the torso, move his hands and finger laterally (outward) without moving his arms (wrist ulnar deviation).

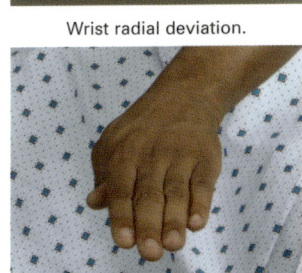

Wrist ulnar deviation.

- Holding his elbows extended in front of his torso, draw imaginary circles with the wrists without moving the arms (wrist circumduction).

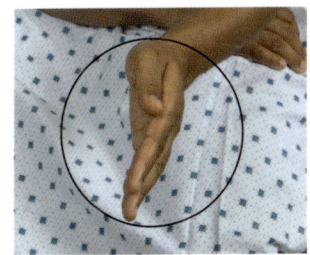

Wrist circumduction.

MUSCULO-SKELETAL

Expected Report

■ Moves wrists through supination, pronation, flexion, extension, radial deviation, ulnar deviation, and circumduction with ease and without crepitus

Assessing the Fingers

Inspection

Ask patient to:

■ Curl his fingers to make a fist (finger flexion).

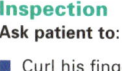

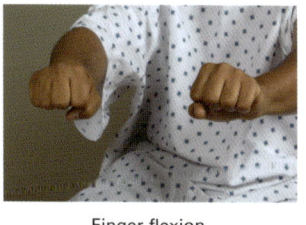

Finger flexion.

■ Open his hands to straighten his fingers (finger extension).

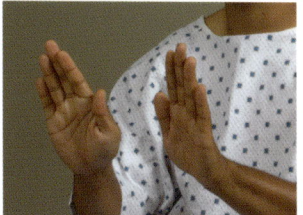

Finger extension.

■ Move all his fingers toward his middle finger (finger adduction).

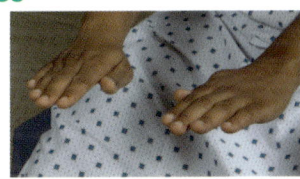

Finger adduction.

■ Move all his fingers away from his middle finger (finger abduction).

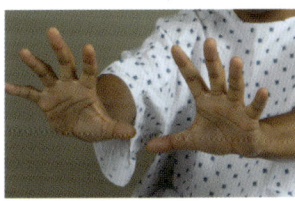

Finger abduction.

Expected Report
■ Moves fingers through flexion, extension, adduction, and abduction with ease and without crepitus

MUSCULO-SKELETAL

Assessing the Spine

Inspection
Ask patient to:

- Bend forward (spine flexion).

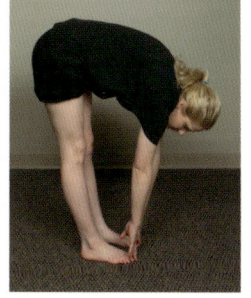

Spine flexion.

- Bend laterally, moving his right hand down the side of his right leg and then his left hand down the side of his left leg (spine lateral flexion).

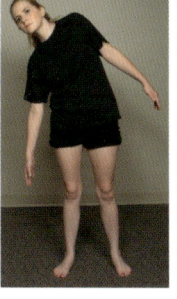 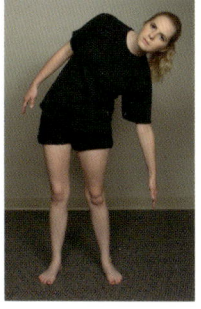

Spine lateral flexion.   Spine lateral flexion.

■ Lean backward (spine extension).

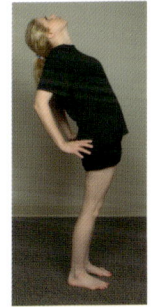

Spine extension.

■ Turn his upper body to the left and then to the right while his feet are in anatomical position (spine rotation).

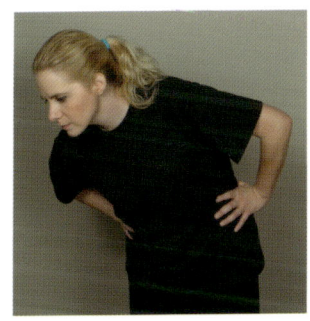

Spine rotation.

Expected Report

■ Moves spine through flexion, lateral flexion, extension, and rotation with ease and without crepitus

Assessing the Hips

Inspection

Ask patient to stand while holding onto the back of a chair or other stable object or to lie supine. Complete ROM assessment is performed on one hip at a time.

Ask patient to:

■ Bring his thigh toward his chest (hip flexion).

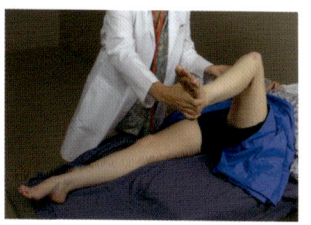

Hip flexion.

■ Move his leg backward, bringing the posterior thigh toward the buttock (hip extension).

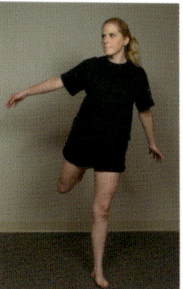

Hip extension.

■ Cross his thigh over the opposite thigh (hip adduction).

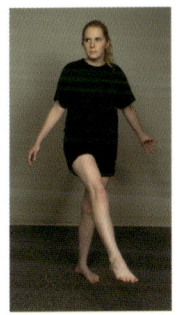

Hip adduction.

■ Lift the thigh up and to the side, away from the midline of the body (hip abduction).

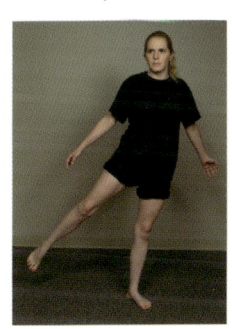

Hip abduction.

MUSCULO-SKELETAL

■ Turn the foot away from the midline of the body (hip lateral rotation).

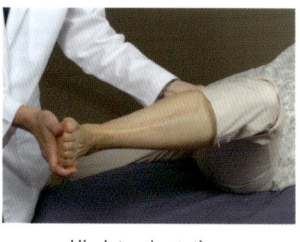

Hip lateral rotation.

■ Turn the foot toward the midline of the body (hip medial rotation).

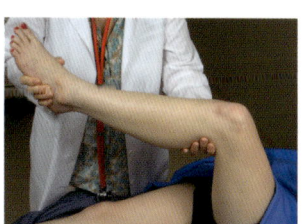

Hip medial rotation.

Expected Report
■ Moves each hip joint through flexion, extension, adduction, abduction, lateral rotation, and medial rotation with ease and without crepitus

Assessing the Knees

Inspection

Ask the patient to stand or to lie supine. Patient may hold onto the back of a chair or other stable object. Complete ROM assessment on one knee at a time.

Ask the patient to:

■ Move his lower leg and foot toward the back of his thigh (knee flexion).

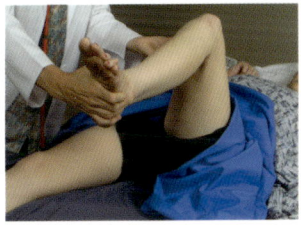

Knee flexion.

■ Hold the leg straight in front of the body (knee extension).

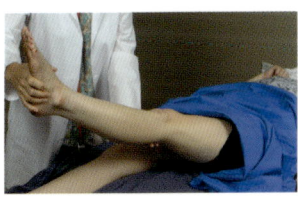

Knee extension.

Expected Report

■ Moves each knee through flexion and extension with ease and without crepitus

Assessing the Ankles

Inspection

Ask the patient to sit with feet off the floor or lie supine. Ask patient to:

- Point his toes toward the floor while lifting his heel upward toward the back of his lower leg (ankle plantar flexion).

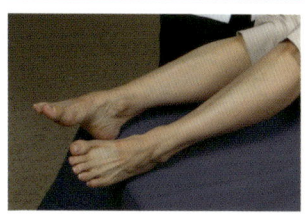

Ankle plantar flexion.

- Point his heel toward the floor while moving toes upward toward shin (ankle dorsiflexion).

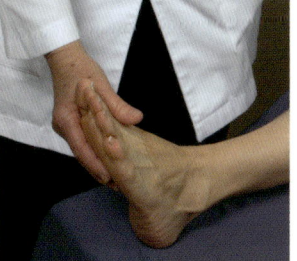

Ankle dorsiflexion.

- Turn the sole of the foot inward (ankle inversion).

Ankle inversion.

- Turn the sole of the foot outward (ankle eversion).

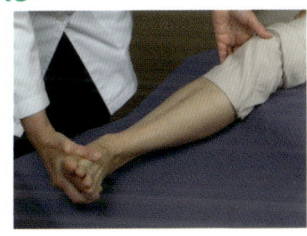

Ankle eversion.

Expected Report
- Moves ankles symmetrically through plantar flexion, dorsi-flexion, inversion, and eversion with ease and without crepitus

Assessing the Toes

Inspection
Ask patient to:

- Curl his toes toward the sole of his foot (toe flexion).

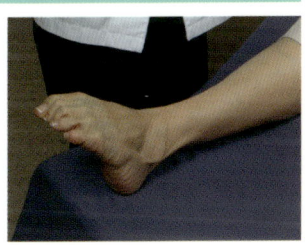

Toe flexion.

- Move his toes toward his shins without moving his foot (toe extension).

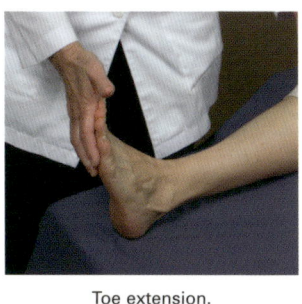

Toe extension.

- Move all his toes toward the middle toe (toe adduction),

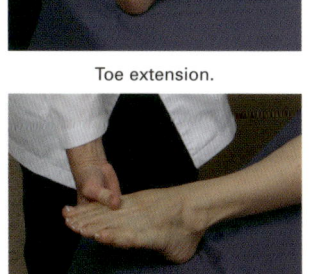

Toe adduction.

- Move all his toes away from his middle toe (toe abduction).

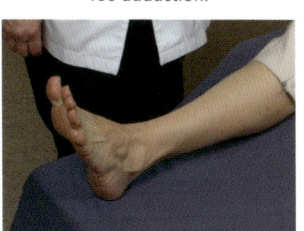

Toe abduction.

Expected Report

■ Moves toes through flexion, extension, adduction, and abduction with ease and without crepitus

Musculoskeletal Assessment Check-Off List

Assessment Task	Performed and Reported Correctly	Performed or Reported Incorrectly	Not Performed
Symmetry, Posture, Alignment, and Equilibrium			
Gross symmetry			
Posture			
Head alignment with shoulders			
Spinal alignment & curves			
Equilibrium (Romberg)			
Gait			
Usual gait			
Tandem heel to toe walk			
Tiptoe walk			
Balance on heels			
Grip			
Upper and Lower Extremity Muscle Strength			
Symmetry and strength of upper extremity medial pushing motion			
Symmetry and strength of upper extremity lateral pushing motion			
Symmetry and strength of upper extremity pulling motion			

Continued

MUSCULO-SKELETAL

Musculoskeletal Assessment Check-Off List—cont'd

Assessment Task	Performed and Reported Correctly	Performed and Reported or Reported Incorrectly	Not Performed
Symmetry and strength of upper extremity anterior pushing motion			
Symmetry and strength of lower extremity pulling motion			
Symmetry and strength of lower extremity pushing motion			
Mobile Joints			
Joints for redness			
Joints for deformity			
Palpation, all mobile joints, warmth			
Palpation, all mobile joints, tenderness			
Temporomandibular Joint (TMJ) ROM			
Protraction			
Retraction			
Extension			
Excursion, lateral			
Cervical Spine (neck) ROM			
Rotation			
Forward flexion			
Extension			
Lateral flexion			
Shoulder ROM			
Flexion			
Extension			

Musculoskeletal Assessment Check-Off List—cont'd

Assessment Task	Performed and Reported Correctly	Performed or Reported Incorrectly	Not Performed
Abduction			
Adduction			
Circumduction			
External rotation			
Internal rotation			
Elbow ROM			
Extension			
Supination			
Pronation			
Flexion			
Wrist ROM			
Supination			
Pronation			
Flexion			
Extension			
Radial deviation			
Ulnar deviation			
Circumduction			
Fingers ROM			
Flexion			
Extension			
Adduction			
Abduction			
Spine ROM			
Flexion			
Lateral flexion			
Extension			
Rotation			

Continued

MUSCULO-SKELETAL

Musculoskeletal Assessment Check-Off List—cont'd

Assessment Task	Performed and Reported Correctly	Performed or Reported Incorrectly	Not Performed
Hip ROM			
Flexion			
Extension			
Adduction			
Abduction			
Lateral rotation			
Medial rotation			
Knee ROM			
Flexion			
Extension			
Ankle ROM			
Plantar flexion			
Dorsiflexion			
Inversion			
Eversion			
Toes ROM			
Flexion			
Extension			
Adduction			
Abduction			

Preparing for the Neurological Assessment

Gather Equipment
- Reflex hammer
- Two paper clips, one opened to expose a sharp tip
- Tongue blade
- Cotton ball or tissue
- Tuning fork, 128 Hz

Prepare Patient
- Explain procedure.
- Patient is standing or seated as appropriate during various parts of the assessment.

Examiner
Stand in front of, behind, or to the side of the patient as needed to assess the neurological system.

Assessing the Neurological System

- Steps in the neurological assessment are often conducted in conjunction with the musculoskeletal assessment.
- Cranial nerves may be tested during the head, ears, eyes, nose, and throat (HEENT) assessment or as part of the neurological exam. Instructions for cranial nerves assessment are integrated into the HEENT & Neck section of this book.

Assessing Proprioception/Cerebellar Function

Inspection
- Ask the patient to sit down.
- To assess rapid alternating movements and coordination:
  - Ask the patient to pat his knees while rapidly supinating (turning palm upward) and pronating (turning palm downward) his open hands.

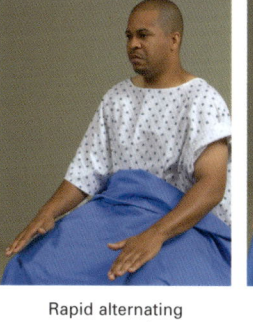

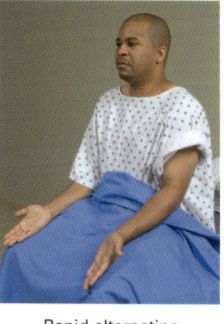

Rapid alternating
movements.

Rapid alternating
movements.

- To assess accuracy of move-
  ment and coordination:
  - Perform the finger-to-finger
    or the precision finger tap
    test by rapidly touching the
    tip of his thumb against
    the tip of each finger on the
    same hand several times,
    beginning with the index fin-
    ger and working toward the
    5th finger, and then repeat-
    ing the process, moving
    from the 5th finger back to
    the index finger.
- To assess coordination:
  - Hold your index finger up about 18 inches from the patient's face.
    Ask the patient to perform the finger-to-nose test by touching his
    nose with his index finger and then moving his finger back and
    forth between his nose and your index finger. Move your finger to
    several different positions during the test.

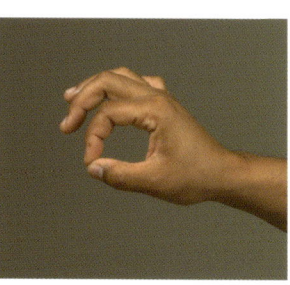

Finger-to-finger test.

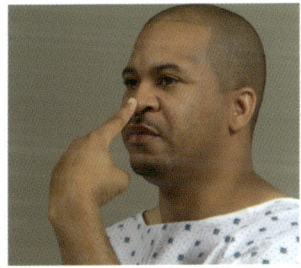

Finger-to-nose test, step 1.

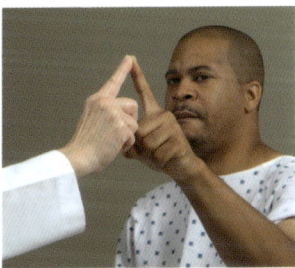

Finger-to-nose test, step 2.

■ Ask the patient to perform the finger-to-nose test with eyes open.

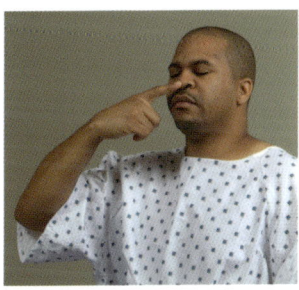

Finger-to-nose test with eyes closed.

- To assess heel-to-shin coordination:
  - Ask the patient to place his right heel against his left shin just under his knee, and then slide his heel down to the top of his left foot, and repeat the motion as quickly as possible without losing heel to shin contact during the downward motion. Repeat the test with the left heel and the right shin.

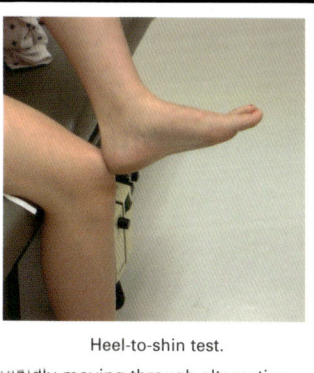

Heel-to-shin test.

Expected Report

- Hands appear coordinated while rapidly moving through alternating supination and pronation of the palms and while quickly moving each fingertip to touch the tip of the thumb on the same hand.
- Movements are accurate with finger-to-nose test with eyes open and with eyes closed.
- Movements are accurate with heel to shin test.
- Coordination is intact.

Unexpected Findings: See p. 181.

Assessing Sensory Function

Inspection

- Ask the patient to sit down and close his or her eyes.
- Assess for stereognosis by placing an object familiar to the patient in his or her hand and asking the patient to identify it.

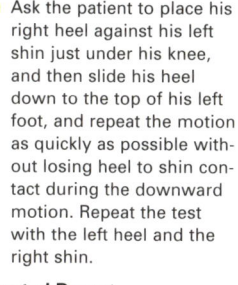

Stereognosis.

- Assess for graphesthesia by asking the patient to identify a number or letter that you draw into the palm of his or her hand with a blunt object.

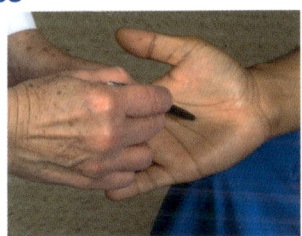

Graphesthesia.

- Assess for perception of superficial touch by asking the patient to identify areas touched as you touch random areas of the body and extremities with a cotton wisp or tissue.

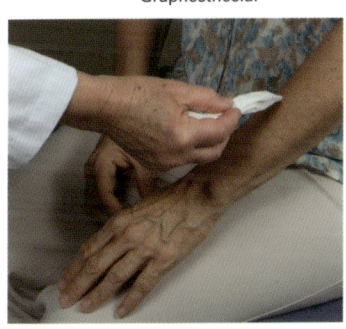

Perception of superficial touch.

- Assess for perception of sharp and dull superficial pain by asking the patient if he or she is being touched with a sharp or dull object as you lightly touch random areas of the body and extremities with the pointed tip of an open paper clip and with the dull curve of a closed paper clip.

Vibratory sensation.

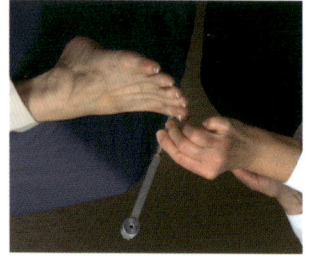

- Assess for perception of vibratory sensation by asking the patient to identify areas touched by an activated tuning fork.

Two point discrimination.

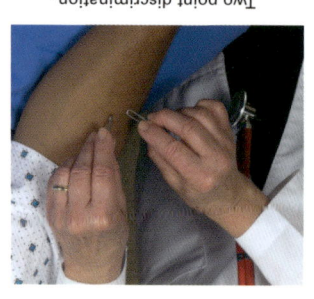

- Assess for two-point discrimination by having the patient tell you whether he or she is being touched by one or two open paper clips as you randomly and lightly touch various areas of the body and extremities with one or two open paper clips.

Perception of sharp.

Perception of dull.

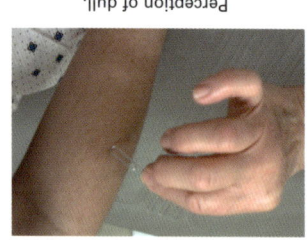

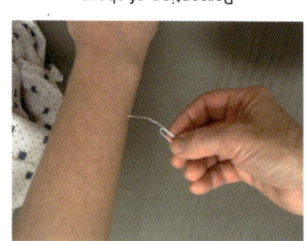

■ Assess for position sense by asking the patient to identify whether digits are being moved to an up or a down position as you move the great toe of each foot and a finger of each hand upward and downward.

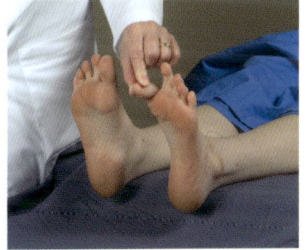

Position sense.

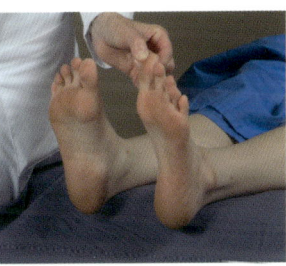

Position sense.

Expected Report
■ Patient identifies familiar object placed into hand while eyes are closed (stereognosis intact).
■ Patient identifies number drawn into the palm of hand while eyes are closed (graphesthesia intact).
■ Patient identifies areas of the body touched with cotton wisp (sensation of superficial touch intact).
■ Patient identifies dull and sharp touch:
  ■ Superficial pain sensation intact.
■ Two-point discrimination intact.
■ Vibratory sensation intact.
■ Position sense intact.

Unexpected Findings: See p. 181.

Assessing Superficial Reflexes

Note that superficial reflexes are a motor response to a scraping motion on the patient's skin.

Plantar or Babinski Reflex

- Ask the patient to sit on the side of the exam table with legs and feet hanging loosely.
- Observe the toes as you use the blunt end of a tongue blade to firmly stroke the lateral side of the plantar surface (sole) of the foot from the heel toward the 5th toe and then moving the tongue blade across the ball of the foot.
  - This test assesses nerve conduction to the spinal levels L4, L5, S1, and S2.

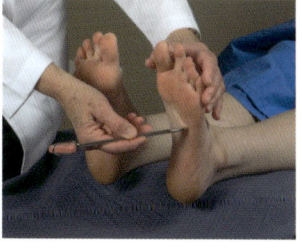

Plantar or Babinski reflex.

Abdominal Reflexes

- The abdominal reflexes are tested as part of the abdominal assessment.
- The abdominal reflexes assess nerve conduction to the spinal levels T7, T8, T9, T10, and T11.

Expected Report

- All toes curl downward in response to stroking the lateral plantar surface and ball of the foot. Plantar reflex normal.

Unexpected Findings: See p. 181.

Assessing Deep Tendon Reflexes

■ Hold the reflex hammer loosely so that it bounces as you briskly tap each deep tendon.

Score deep-tendon movements as follows:

0	No response or absent (areflexia)	Abnormal
1+	Hypoactive response (hyporeflexia)	May or may not be abnormal
2+ or ++	Brisk or expected response	Normal
3+ or +++	Very brisk (hyperreflexia)	May or may not be abnormal
4+ or +++	Very brisk with sustained clonus (sustained series of rapid jerky movements)	Abnormal

Note that some references recommend use of a 5-point grading scale, with 4+ being non-sustained clonus and 5+ being sustained clonus.

Biceps Deep Tendon Reflex

■ Ask the seated patient to place his hands on his thighs, with his elbows semi-flexed.

■ Place the fingers of your non-dominant hand behind his elbow, and place your thumb over the biceps tendon located in the antecubital fossa (inner elbow).

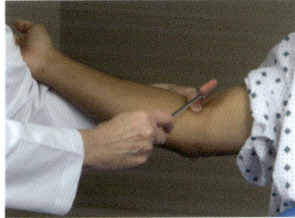

■ Strike your thumb with the reflex hammer.

■ This test assesses spinal nerve root C7.

Biceps reflex.

Expected Report

■ Elbow flexes when biceps tendon is tapped; biceps reflex 2+

Unexpected Findings: See p. 181.

Triceps Deep Tendon Reflex

- Hold the patient's upper arm in your non-dominant hand, with the elbow bent and the lower arm hanging loosely.
- Place the thumb of your non-dominant hand over the triceps tendon.
- Strike your thumb with the reflex hammer.
  - This test assesses spinal nerve roots C7 and C8.

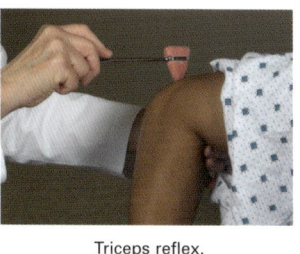

Triceps reflex.

Expected Report

- Elbow extends when triceps tendon is tapped; triceps reflex 2+

Unexpected Findings: See p. 181.

Brachioradialis Deep Tendon Reflex

- Support the patient's wrist and lower arm with your non-dominant hand.
- Place your thumb over the brachioradialis area tendon, which is about 1 cm lateral and about 8 cm above the usual site of radial pulse assessment.
- Strike your thumb with the reflex hammer.
- This reflex may also be tested directly by tapping the tendon.
  - This test assesses spinal nerve roots C6 and C7.

Brachioradialis reflex.

Expected Report

- Elbow flexes when brachioradialis tendon is tapped; brachioradialis reflex 2+

Unexpected Findings: See p. 181.

Patellar or Knee Jerk Deep Tendon Reflex

■ Ask the patient to sit on the side of the exam table with legs hanging freely.

■ Tap the patellar tendon in the space between the patella and the tibial tuberosity.

  ■ This test assesses spinal nerve roots L 3 to L5.

  ■ Note that if lower extremity deep tendon reflexes (DTR) are difficult to elicit, responses may be intensified or augmented by asking the patient to curl the fingers of both hands and use the curled fingers of each hand to grasp and pull tightly on the curled fingers of the opposite hand. This maneuver is called "augmentation" of the reflex response.

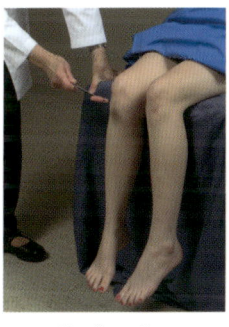

Patellar reflex.

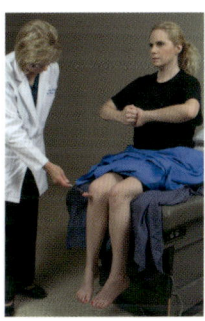

Augmentation of lower extremity DTR responses.

Expected Report

■ Knee extends when patellar tendon tapped

■ Patellar reflexes 2+

Unexpected Findings: See p. 181.

Unexpected Findings: See p. 181.

NEURO

Ankle Jerk Reflex (Achilles Reflex or Ankle Clonus)

- Also known as the clonus reflex and the Achilles reflex
- Ask patient to sit on exam table with legs hanging freely
- Place your hand under sole of his foot and gently dorsi-flex (push backwards) distal foot
- Tap Achilles tendon just above its calcaneal insertion (just superior to the heel)
  - Assesses spinal nerve roots S1 and S2

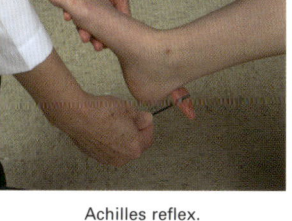

Achilles reflex.

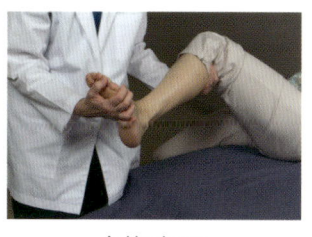

Ankle clonus.

Expected Report

- Distal foot plantar-flexes when Achilles tendon tapped
- Achilles reflex 2+

Unexpected Findings: See p. 181.

Neurological Assessment Check-Off List

Assessment Task	Performed and Recorded Correctly	Performed or Reported Incorrectly	Not Performed
Rapid alternating movements			
Finger-to-finger test			
Finger-to-nose test			
Finger-to-nose test (eyes closed)			
Heel-to-shin test			
Stereognosis			
Graphesthesia			
Superficial touch			
Sharp vs. dull perception			
Two-point discrimination			
Vibratory sense			
Position sense			
Plantar or Babinski reflex			
Biceps DTR			
Triceps DTR			
Brachioradialis DTR			
Patellar DTR			
Ankle jerk DTR			
Ankle clonus			

Unexpected Findings

Mental Status

Level of Consciousness
- Lack of appropriate response to verbal, visual, or tactile stimuli may indicate mental illness or brain disorder.

Appearance, Posture, and Grooming
- Unkempt appearance; dirty or inappropriately dressed for gender, season, or occasion; or slumped posture may indicate depression or brain disorder.

Orientation to Time, Person, and Place
- Inability to identify current date, own name, or current location indicates mental illness or brain disorder.

Mood/Affect/Behavior
- Sad or apathetic expression may indicate depression.
- Fixed, immobile features may indicate Parkinsonism.
- Fearful expression may indicate anxiety, disorientation, or mental illness.

Concentration/Attention Span
- Inability to focus attention enough to adequately cooperate with the physical exam process, or asking for questions to be repeated in the absence of a hearing problem may indicate anxiety, mental illness, or attention deficit disorder.

Memory (Immediate, Short-Term, Long-Term, or Remote)
- Inability to answer memory questions correctly may indicate mental retardation or mental illness.

Abstract Thinking
- Patient responds by providing a concrete (rather than abstract or comparison to a life situation) explanation of a proverb or metaphor, fails to provide any explanation for a metaphor or proverb.
- May indicate lack of intelligence, dementia, brain damage, or psychosis

Analogies
- Inability to compare items correctly may indicate lack of intelligence or brain damage.

Judgment
- Failure to respond appropriately may indicate lack of intelligence, brain disease, or psychosis.

Calculation
- Failure to correctly respond to simple calculation questions may indicate lack of intelligence, brain disease, or depression.

Integumentary

Skin
- **Pallor** (paleness) may indicate anemia or poor tissue perfusion. Poor tissue perfusion may be caused by a cardiovascular condition or cold environmental temperature.
- **Cyanosis** (bluish color) may indicate lack of oxygenation that is cardiac or respiratory in origin.
- **Jaundice** (yellowish tint) may indicate hemolysis (breakdown of red blood cells due to sickle cell disease or other conditions) or liver disease such as hepatitis.
- Isolated pallor, cyanosis, or erythema of isolated areas, such as fingers, toes, earlobes, or nose, may indicate Raynaud's disease or phenomenon.
- Malodorous skin may indicate infection, lack of appropriate personal hygiene due to homelessness or mental illness, or a metabolic disorder.
- Skin that feels hot to the touch may indicate fever, localized inflammation, or infection of the site being touched.
- Skin that feels cold to the touch may indicate poor circulation or cold exposure.
- Dry skin may indicate dehydration or thyroid disorder.
- Coarse skin may indicate repeated trauma.
- Slow skin recoil during skin turgor assessment is a late sign of dehydration.

Lesions

- Skin breakdown or open lesion in the skin indicates a history of surgery, trauma, or inflammation.
- Individual lesions should be described in the following manner:
  - Shape
  - Size (measure with centimeter ruler)
  - Intact or open surface
  - Texture appearance if surface is intact
  - Depressed, flat, or elevated
    - Remember: "You can pat a papule, and a macule looks mashed."
  - Color
  - Drainage (report amount, color, consistency)
  - Exact location

Types of Skin Lesions

Macule: flat, less than 1 cm
Papule: elevated, firm, less than 1 cm
Nodule: elevated, firm, 1 to 2 cm
Tumor: elevated, firm, greater than 2 cm
Plaque: firm, rough top, greater than 1 cm
Vesicle: elevated, superficial, filled with clear liquid, less than 1 cm
Cyst: elevated, deeper than vesicle, filled with liquid or soft matter
Pustule: elevated, filled with purulent liquid
Fissure: linear crack in skin

- A **mole** that is larger and/or looks different from the majority of moles on a patient may indicate pathology.
- A mole that has any one of following characteristics may indicate skin cancer:
  - **A**—Asymmetry of lesion
  - **B**—Border irregularity
  - **C**—Color: multiple colors in a lesion
  - **D**—Diameter over 6 mm (size of pencil eraser)
  - **E**—Evolving, changing in size, color, or shape

Groups of Lesions

- A group or groups of similar lesions may indicate skin pathology, such as molluscum contagiosum lesions (a virus) or a systemic condition such as herpes zoster (chickenpox) or measles.

- Groups of similar skin lesions are described in the following manner:
  - Pattern or configuration of group such as linear or serpentine
  - Discrete (lesions not touching each other) or confluent (running together)
  - Color or colors of lesions and surrounding skin
  - Secondary lesion changes, such as crusting
  - Drainage; report amount, color, consistency
  - Location on body (location may be described as "generalized" if similar lesions cover the entire body)

Scalp
- Dirty scalp may indicate poor hygiene or physical or mental disability.
- Lesions may indicate local or systemic disorder.
- Parasites may indicate poor hygiene or exposure to a common parasite source such as a wooded area or a densely populated environment.

Hair
- Dirty hair may indicate homelessness, substance abuse, mental illness, or retardation.
- Reddish brown color with excessive broken hair strands may indicate malnutrition.
- Symmetrical hair loss may indicate thyroid disorder.
- Asymmetrical bald areas may indicate local infection, abuse, or self hair-pulling related to mental illness.
- Coarse hair may indicate hypothyroidism.
- Fine hair may indicate hyperthyroidism.
- Broken or easily broken strands of hair may indicate thyroid disorder.

Nails
- Rounded nails (clubbing) may indicate chronic lung or heart disease.
- Concave-shaped nails (spoon nails) may indicate chronic anemia.
- Dirty nails may indicate poor hygiene or physical or mental disability.
- Transverse indentations (Beau's lines) may indicate a history of acute severe illness, surgery, chronic eczema, or stress. Transverse indentation on a single nail indicates injury of the specific nail.
- Thick, yellow, or dark-colored nails may indicate nail fungus (onychomycosis).
- Spongy feeling due to weak attachment to nailbed may indicate chronic local infection.
- Nailbed attachment angle of greater than 180° is seen in clubbing, which may indicate chronic lung or heart disease.

Head, Eyes, Ears, Nose, Throat, and Neck

Head
- Hydrocephaly is an enlarged head caused by failure of spinal fluid to circulate or reabsorb.
- Microcephaly is a small head that may be genetic or due to mental retardation.
- Asymmetry of the head may be due to surgery or injury.
- Scaling, masses, or tenderness of scalp may indicate infection or tumor.
- Lumps, bumps, tenderness, lesions, and scars may be caused by traumatic injury, infection, or parasitic infection.

Face
- Asymmetry of facial features may indicate cardiovascular accident (CVA) (stroke) or cranial nerve injury.
- Sad or fixed expression may indicate depression.
- Expressionless face may accompany depression or Parkinson's disease.
- Tense or frowning expression may indicate confusion, anxiety, anger, or depression.
- **CN V, Trigeminal:** Weak or asymmetrical contractions *of the temporal and masseter muscles* may be due to a musculoskeletal or a neurological disorder.
- **CN V, Trigeminal Motor:** Absent corneal blink reflex may be caused by an injury or a lesion of cranial nerve V or VII or may be associated with herpes simplex infection.
- **CN VII, Facial:** Weakness or asymmetry of facial movements may indicate CVA (stroke) or cranial nerve injury; involuntary movements may indicate a tic or tardive dyskinesia or may be psychogenic.

Eyes
Eyebrows and Lashes
- Absent brows or lashes may be the result of chemotherapy or intentional pulling.
- Absence of lateral portion of eyebrows may indicate hypothyroidism (Hertzoge's sign).
- Eyelashes turned inward, such as occurs with entropion (turning inward of eyelids), causes eye discomfort and may result in corneal damage.

166

Eyelids and Lacrimal Apparatus

- Swelling or blepharitis (inflammation) may be the result of irritation, allergy, or infection.
- Lesions may be caused by trauma, infection, or cancer.
- Ectropion (lid eversion) may occur with muscle weakness, aging, or rapid weight loss.
- Entropion (lid inversion) may be due to muscle loss with aging or may be due to scarring.
- Unilateral ptosis (dropping of the eyelid) may be caused by weakness of a muscle, damage to the sympathetic nervous system (Horner syndrome), or birth defect.
- Bilateral ptosis may be caused by CVA (stroke) or myasthenia gravis.
- Lesions may be hordeolum or stye, an infection of sebaceous gland or chalazion, a blocked sebaceous gland, or xanthelasma; a yellowish plaque on the eyelids that may indicate elevated cholesterol.
- Swelling, tenderness, redness of lacrimal apparatus may indicate blockage and/or infection.
- Excess tears or purulent drainage from lacrimal apparatus may indicate irritation, allergy, or infection.

Globe of Eye

- Protrusion of globe of eye may be genetic or may be associated with hyperthyroidism (if bilateral) or tumor (if unilateral)

Conjunctiva

- Red conjunctiva may indicate irritation, allergy, or infection.
- Pale conjunctiva may indicate anemia.
- Dry conjunctiva may indicate dehydration or autoimmune disease such as Sjögren's disease.

Sclera, Iris, Cornea, and Lens

- Sclera "injected" (red) or with visible hemorrhage may be caused by injury or severe cough.
- Pterygium, a lesion of thin tissue, is usually on the nasal side of the eye and is more common in those who are exposed to ultraviolet light.
- Coloboma is a congenital defect that may appear as a dark hole or notch in the iris of the eye.
- Cloudy cornea may be caused by nutritional deficiency, infection, or Sjögren's disease.

UNEXP-
FINDS

■ Arcus senilis is a thin, grayish circle at the edge of the cornea. It appears to encircle the iris and may be benign or an indication of hyperlipidemia.

■ Cataract (clouding of the lens) gives the pupil a foggy appearance and impairs vision.

Corneal Light Reflex and Cover-Uncover Test

■ An asymmetrical corneal light reflex or a positive cover-uncover test may indicate strabismus.
  ■ **NOTE:** patient with positive cover-uncover test should be referred to an eye care professional.

■ **CN III, Oculomotor; CN IV, Trochlear; CN VI Abducens:**
  ■ **Pupillary Light Reflex and Accommodation:** Pupil size and reactivity to direct and indirect light or examiner's finger position changes may indicate CN III damage, drugs, tumors, diabetes, other systemic diseases, and brain death or hypoxia.
  ■ **Convergence:** Marked nystagmus or uncoordinated eye movements may be related to a CNS disorder, metabolic disease, or drug or alcohol intoxication.

■ **CN II, Optic:**
  ■ Inability to read the 20/20 line on a Snellen or other standard chart may indicate myopia or nearsightedness and should be evaluated by an eye care professional.
  ■ Inability of a young adult to read newsprint or the 20/20 line on a Rosenbaum chart without corrective lenses may indicate hyperopia, known as farsightedness, and should be evaluated by an eye care professional.
  ■ Inability of an adult over the age of 30 to read the newspaper or the Rosenbaum 20/20 line may indicate presbyopia, the result of age-related loss of lens flexibility.
  ■ **Confrontation Test:**
    • Visual fields or peripheral vision that is not equal to that of the examiner may indicate glaucoma.
  ■ **Retinal or Fundoscopic Exam:**
    • Absence of red reflex, swollen edges of optic disk, or cup-disk ratio less than 0.3, AV nicking, hemorrhages, copper wiring, or cotton wool may indicate a disease such as hypertension or diabetes.

- A swollen optic disk may indicate brain swelling.
- Note that the location of any abnormality is reported in disk diameters from the optic disk and by referring to clock face positions, such as "exudate is noted two disk diameters from the optic disk at the 2 o'clock position."

Nose

- Asymmetry of nose or deviated septum may indicate injury or deformity.
- Perforation of septum may indicate cocaine use or injury.
- Red mucosa may indicate infection or traumatic irritation.
- Pale mucosa may indicate anemia or allergy.
- Bluish mucosa may indicate allergy.
- Swollen or reddened turbinates may indicate upper respiratory infection, allergic rhinitis, vasomotor rhinitis, a drug reaction, or hormonal influence.
- Polyps grow from the lining of the nose and may be seen in patients with chronic conditions such as cystic fibrosis, asthma, or allergic rhinitis, or who have aspirin sensitivity.
- Note that although swollen turbinates and polyps may appear similar, swollen turbinates are usually painful, whereas polyps are not painful.
    - **CN I, Olfactory:**
        - Anosmia (loss of the sense of smell) may be inherited or related to a brain tumor, atherosclerosis, rhinitis, sinusitis, smoking, zinc deficiency, or cocaine use.
        - The common cold is the most frequent cause of loss of the sense of smell.

Sinuses

- Absence of observable light in the mouth upon transillumination of the sinuses may indicate sinus infection or an abnormal growth in the sinus.
- Tenderness over a sinus cavity may indicate irritation or infection.
- Note that the patient may report food having "lost its taste" when the sense of smell is deficient.

Mouth
Lips
- Dry, cracked lips may indicate dehydration or mouth breathing and are more common in dry climates.
- Lip lesions may be caused by herpesvirus (cold sores), irritation, or traumatic injury.
- Chelar fissures (cracking of skin in the corners of the mouth) may be caused by a fungal infection, vitamin B deficiency, or chemical irritation.
- Deep fissure in upper lip is consistent with cleft lip, a congenital disorder.

Teeth
- Broken teeth or jagged edges
- Caries (decay)
- Severe underbite or overbite may result in malocclusion or temporomandibular joint problems

Oral Mucosa and Gums
- *Pallor* (paleness) of mucosa membranes may indicate anemia or poor tissue perfusion.
- Bluish tint may indicate cyanosis.
- Lesions of oral mucosa may be caused by infection including candida infection (thrush); carcinoma, trauma, or ill-fitting or jagged teeth.
- Red or receding or bleeding gums may be a sign of gingivitis (gum disease), which leads to tooth loss.

Salivary Glands
- Swelling of salivary glands may indicate infection, tumor, or sialolithiasis (salivary gland stones).

Tongue
- Ulcers or other lesions on tongue may indicate allergy or infection.
- Black or furry coating on posterior tongue may indicate tobacco use, poor hygiene, antibiotic use, or recent bismuth subsalicylate (such as Pepto-Bismol) use.
- *CN XII, Hypoglossal:* Weakness or tremors of the tongue may indicate a motor neuron disease such as amyotrophic lateral sclerosis.

- **CN IX, Glossopharyngeal, and CN X, Vagus:**
  - Inability to identify taste may indicate decrease in number of taste buds, which occurs with occluded nasal passage.
    - Note that loss of ability to smell results in decreased sense of taste.
  - Failure of the uvula to rise in midline may indicate scar tissue or a tumor of CN X.
  - Loss of ability to swallow or speak may indicate that a CVA (stroke) has occurred.

Pharynx and Tonsils

- Fissure in or discontinuous palate is consistent with cleft palate.
- Red pharynx or red and swollen tonsils may indicate infection.
- Enlarged tonsils with white or gray exudate may indicate infection.
- Purulent drainage in posterior pharynx may indicate viral or bacterial infection.
- Uvula deviation may be related to a tumor of the vagus nerve, scar tissue, or scoliosis.

Ear

Outer Ear

- Tops of ears set lower than the inner canthus of the eye is a common finding in mental retardation.
- The outer ear is a common site for seborrhea and cancerous lesions.
- Tophi (deposits of urate crystals) may indicate gout.
- **CN VIII, Vestibulocochlear or Acoustic:**
  - **Gross Hearing Test, Whisper Test:** Failure to identify whispered words may indicate conductive or sensorineural hearing loss.
  - **Weber Test:** With conductive hearing loss, sound is louder (localizes) in deficient ear. With sensorineural hearing loss, sound is louder (localizes) toward the good ear.
  - **Rinne Test:** With conductive hearing loss, bone conduction is longer than or equal to air conduction. Conductive hearing loss is caused by an obstruction such as cerumen impaction or otitis media. With sensorineural hearing loss, air conduction is longer than bone conduction, but the ratio is less than 2:1. Sensorineural hearing loss is the result of nerve damage.
  - **Vestibular Test:** Eyes that move in the same direction as the turned head indicate brainstem disorder.

Ear Canal
- Red, swollen canals or drainage may indicate infection (otitis externa).
- Excess cerumen may cause conductive hearing loss.
- Foreign bodies, such as insects or peas in the ear canal, may cause impaired hearing, pain, trauma, or infection.

Tympanic Membrane (TM)
- Red or bulging TM may indicate infection. Acute infection of the TM is known as acute otitis media (AOM).
- Fever may cause the TM to appear red.
- Absent or interrupted light reflex in the absence of bulging of the TM may indicate TM retraction caused by otitis media with effusion (OME), also known as serous otitis media (SOM).
- Retraction of the TM causes bony landmarks to appear more prominent.
- Bulging of the TM may result in disappearance of bony landmarks.
- **CN XI, Spinal Accessory:**
  - Weakness of muscles may indicate a CVA (stroke)

Neck
Lymph Nodes of Head and Neck
- Swelling of nodes or redness over nodes may indicate infection. These nodes are mobile.
- Fixed, non-mobile nodes that are generally non-tender may be attached to an underlying tumor.

Thyroid
- Enlargement of thyroid tissue is called goiter and may accompany hypothyroidism or hyperthyroidism.
- Masses or small lumps in thyroid tissue may be benign or malignant.

Chest and Breasts

Anterior and Axillary Chest
Inspection
- Lesions may indicate infection, birthmarks, moles, or injury. Petechial lesions may indicate pulmonary embolism.
- Scars indicate past surgery, injury, or infection.

- Asymmetry of the chest may indicate trauma, past surgical procedures, or genetic deformity.
- Rapid respirations (tachypnea) may indicate hypoxia, anxiety, pneumonia asthma, chronic obstructive pulmonary disease (COPD), or shock.
- Shallow respirations may indicate anxiety, asthma, pulmonary edema, shock, pneumonia, or hyperventilation.
- Slow respirations (bradypnea) may indicate sedation, brain damage, or respiratory fatigue.
- A prolonged expiratory phase may indicate trapped air such as occurs with asthma or COPD.
- Irregular respiratory rhythm may have numerous causes including embolism, drug abuse, poisoning, or a brain injury or disorder.
- Deep and labored breathing may indicate acidosis such as occurs with diabetic ketoacidosis or renal failure.
- A costal angle greater than 90° may be caused by hyperinflation of the lungs such as occurs with COPD.

Palpation
- Palpation of masses may indicate tumors, sebaceous cysts, genetic deformity, or fractures.
- Crepitus, also called subcutaneous emphysema, indicates trapped air beneath the skin and may be caused by a penetrating chest or abdominal wound, tuberculosis, emphysema, esophageal rupture, infection, or pneumothorax.
- Increased tactile fremitus is caused by the presence of consolidation, fluids, or solids.
- Decreased tactile fremitus is caused by excess air in the lungs such as occurs with pleural effusion, pneumothorax, or COPD.
- Asymmetrical respiratory excursion may indicate numerous lung or abdominal pathologies, including asthma, COPD, or heart disease.

Percussion
- Dullness over the lung fields may indicate a tumor or fluid in the lungs such as occurs with pneumonia or pleural effusion.
- Hyperresonance indicates a condition that results in excess air in the lungs such as COPD, asthma, or pneumothorax.
- Tympany, a drum-like sound, may indicate pneumothorax.

Auscultation

- Bronchial sounds auscultated over the peripheral lung fields may indicate consolidation such as occurs with pneumonia or pulmonary edema.
- Rales, a crackling sound, may indicate pneumonia.
- Rhonchi, a coarse, snoring-like sound, may be heard with COPD, asthma, or bronchitis.
- Wheezing, a musical sound, indicates decreased size of the airway lumens and is usually heard during expiration or early inspiration; it may indicate asthma, pneumonia, bronchitis, or other conditions.

Posterior Chest

Inspection
See Anterior and Axillary Chest.

Palpation
See Anterior and Axillary Chest

Percussion

- Decreased diaphragmatic excursion may indicate bronchitis, pleural effusion, atelectasis, COPD, pneumothorax, asthma, or pneumonia.
- Bronchophony is heard as a loud, clear sound as the patient says "99" and may indicate lung cancer or fluid in the lungs, such as occurs with pneumonia.

Auscultation

- Whispered pectoriloquy is heard as clearly whispered words as the patient says "99" and may indicate cancer or fluid in the lungs, such as occurs with pneumonia.
- Egophony is heard as "ay" when the patient says "ee" and may indicate cancer, pneumonia, or fibrosis.

Breasts

- Marked asymmetry of the breasts may indicate a tumor or mastitis.
- Lesions may indicate trauma, infection, or cancer.
- Puckering or "orange peel"–appearing skin may indicate cancer.
- Markedly small breast size may indicate malnutrition or a hormone abnormality.
- Increased breast size in males and females may indicate mastitis, tumors, marijuana use, hormone abnormality, or numerous medications.

- Nipple inversion may be genetic or may be the result of breastfeeding or cancer.
- Masses may indicate infection, fibrocystic disease, or cancer.

Cardiovascular

Peripheral Circulation
Edema
- Edema may indicate heart failure or renal disease.

Color
- Pallor (paleness) may indicate anemia or poor tissue perfusion.
  - Poor tissue perfusion may be caused by a cardiovascular condition such as heart failure or cold environmental temperature.
- Cyanosis (bluish color) may indicate lack of oxygenation that is cardiac or respiratory in origin.
- Isolated pallor or cyanosis of any digits (fingers or toes), earlobes, or nose may indicate Raynaud's disease/phenomenon or a blocked artery.
- Erythema of a digit may indicate Raynaud's disease or phenomenon or inflammation.
  - **Raynaud's phenomenon** may be linked to autoimmune conditions such as Lupus.
  - **Raynaud's disease** is not associated with an autoimmune condition.
  - Both Raynaud's disease and phenomenon are caused by *arteriole spasms*.

Capillary Refill
- Nail capillary refill that takes longer than 2 seconds may be caused by impaired blood flow to the digit.

Peripheral Pulses
Amplitude or Strength
- Pulses difficult to palpate or absent or increased pulse strength.
- Weak pulses may be caused by low blood pressure, hemorrhage, shock, dehydration, or heart failure.

Heart Rate and Rhythm
- Absent pulses may be caused by cardiac arrest or arterial occlusion.
- Increased pulse strength may be caused by elevated blood pressure, anemia, fever, or thyrotoxicosis.

- A sustained pulse rate higher than 100 beats per minute is known as tachycardia. Some causes are anemia, fever, emotions, shock, or medications.
- A sustained pulse rate lower than 60 beats per minute is known as bradycardia. Some causes are hypothyroidism, heart disease or defect, electrolyte imbalance, or medications such as beta blockers.
- An irregular pulse may be caused by heart disease or defect, electrolyte imbalance, head injury, or excess caffeine.

Pulse Deficit

- A pulse deficit, with the apical pulse being higher than the radial pulse, may be caused by circulatory problems or atrial fibrillation.

Temporal Arteries

- Bruit(s) heard over temporal arteries may indicate partially occluded arteries.

Carotid Arteries

- Bruit heard in either or both carotid arteries indicates partial obstruction.

Precordium

Inspection

- Lesions may indicate injury, irritation, eczema, allergy, or infection.
- Scars indicate past surgery or other trauma.
- An apical impulse or point of maximum impulse (PMI) that exceeds 3 cm in diameter may indicate a displaced or enlarged heart.
- An apical impulse or PMI that is displaced laterally may indicate a past infarct.

Palpation

- An exaggerated apical impulse may indicate left increased cardiac output, left ventricular hypertrophy, or hyperthyroidism and is called a lift or heave, with a heave being more forceful than a lift.
- A thrill is a palpable vibratory sensation caused by turbulent blood flow and is associated with a heart murmur that is grade IV, V, or VI.

Heart Sounds

- S_3 occurs immediately after S_2 in early diastole when the ventricles are filling. It may indicate early heart failure, mitral or aortic regurgitation, or fluid volume overload.

■ S_4 occurs in late diastole, just before S_1, and may indicate hypertension, pulmonary hypertension, cardiomyopathies, or pulmonic or aortic stenosis.

Murmurs

Murmurs are described and reported according to:

■ Timing and duration
  ■ Systolic (early or late systole)
  ■ Diastolic
■ Location heard best
  ■ Aortic
  ■ Pulmonic
  ■ Tricuspid
  ■ Mitral
■ Intensity (loudness)
  ■ I/VI = barely audible
  ■ II/VI = soft but audible after a few seconds
  ■ III/VI = moderately loud and easy to hear
  ■ IV/VI = loud and thrill may be felt
  ■ V/VI = heard with stethoscope half way off the chest and thrill easily felt
  ■ VI/VI = heard with stethoscope completely off the chest and with thrill easily felt
■ Pitch
  ■ High or low
■ Radiation

Friction Rub

■ A friction rub is caused by an inflamed pericardia sac, lasts through systole and diastole, and overlies other cardiac sounds.

Jugular Veins

Inspection (Jugular Venous Pressure (JVP), Patient at 45° Angle)

■ JVP above 8 cm may indicate fluid volume overload or right-sided heart failure.
■ JVP below 5 may indicate hypovolemia.

Percussion (Heart, Patient in Left Lateral Recumbent Position)

■ Lateral corner of cardiac dullness (LBCD) that is displaced to the left may indicate old cardiac infarct and cardiac enlargement.

Auscultation (Heart, Patient in Left Lateral Recumbent Position or Supine Position)

■ Refer to preceding bullet for interpretation of abnormal auscultation findings.

Abdomen

Inspection
Symmetry

■ Asymmetry may indicate abnormal growth(s) or obstruction.

Skin Color

■ Reddened (erythematous) skin may indicate fever, inflammation, or infection.
■ Pallor (paleness) of skin may indicate anemia or poor tissue perfusion.
■ Blue tint to skin may indicate cyanosis.

Scars

■ Scars are related to past trauma that may have been caused by surgery, infection, inflammation, or wounds induced by accidental or intentional actions.
■ Striae are silvery lines caused by past stretching of the skin that was followed by weight loss; often seen following pregnancy or Cushing's disease.

Lesions

■ Lesions may indicate benign nevi or birthmarks, skin cancer, inflammation, allergy, trauma, or infection that is either local or systemic.
■ Bulging flanks (areas between the lowest rib and the upper edge of the hip bone) may indicate *ascites* (collection of fluid in the abdominal cavity, known as the peritoneal cavity) and is usually the result of severe liver disease or cirrhosis.

Abdominal Contour

■ A protuberant abdomen indicates ascites, infection, obstruction, or obesity.
■ A severely sunken abdomen is called a scaphoid abdomen and may indicate malnutrition, dehydration, or diaphragmatic hernia.

178

Umbilicus
- A swollen or markedly protruding umbilicus may indicate inflammation, infection, a growth, or an umbilical hernia.
- Superficial bruising and edema around the umbilicus may indicate ruptured ectopic pregnancy or pancreatitis and is called Cullen's sign.

Patient Supine
- Visible peristalsis may indicate intestinal obstruction that is the result of a growth, a hernia, intestinal malrotation, stenosis, fecal impaction, or inflammation.
- Marked pulsation over the aorta may indicate aneurysm.
- Bulging or masses in specific areas may indicate a tumor or hernia.
- Enlarged veins may indicate a blood vessel disorder, tumor, cancer, or acute pancreatitis or may accompany ascites.

Auscultation—Using Stethoscope's Bell
- A bruit is an arterial sound that is similar to the sound of liquid being forced through a small opening or similar to a breath sound. A bruit is caused by a stenosed or partially occluded artery or by a high volume of blood rushing through an artery.
- A friction rub indicates inflammation of the organ. It is high-pitched, and timing can be anticipated by watching respiratory movement.

Auscultation—Using Stethoscope's Diaphragm
- Loud and prolonged bowel sounds are called borborygmi and may be caused by gastrointestinal infection, early obstruction, or hunger.
- Very high-pitched bowel sounds may occur with early obstruction.
- Decreased or absent bowel sounds may be caused by peritonitis or paralytic ileus.

Percussion
- A dull percussion note in any unexpected area may indicate organ enlargement and disease, tumor, or an area of fecal-filled colon.

Palpation
- Palpation of a mass in any unexpected area may indicate organ enlargement and disease, tumor, or an area of fecal-filled colon.

Superficial Abdominal Reflexes
- Ipsilateral (same side) abdominal reflexes may be absent in the patient with a corticospinal tract lesion.

Inguinal Lymph Nodes
- Enlarged lymph nodes may indicate infection of the legs, feet, or pelvic area or may indicate allergy or malignancy.

Musculoskeletal

Symmetry, Posture, Alignment, and Equilibrium
- Asymmetry of the torso or individual body parts may indicate birth defect, injury, muscle atrophy, scoliosis, or a CVA.
- Slumped posture may indicate poor muscle tone, osteopenia, osteoporosis, pain, fatigue, or depression.
- Malalignment of the head may indicate nerve or muscle injury, birth defect, pain, scoliosis, or poor vision.
- Malalignment of the spine may indicate scoliosis, nerve damage, osteoporosis, or pain.
- A positive Romberg test may indicate intoxication or a vestibular, cerebellar, or spinal disorder.

Gait
- An abnormal gait, inaccurate tandem toe walk, or tiptoe walk or heel balance may indicate intoxication, pain, or a muscular or nervous system disorder.

Upper and Lower Extremity Muscle Strength
- Weakness of pushing or pulling motions in the upper or lower extremities or asymmetrical strength may indicate a bone, muscle, tendon, or ligament disorder or may indicate a neurological disorder, such as that of a spinal nerve root.

Mobile Joints
Inspection
- Redness of a joint may be caused by an inflammatory process, gout, or infection.
- Deformity of a joint may be caused by a birth defect, injury, or an inflammatory or degenerative process.
- Crepitus of a joint may be caused by arthritis or infection.
- Asymmetry of joint movement may be caused by pain, joint inflammation, or infection.
- Limited range of joint motion may be caused by injury, arthritis, inflammation, or muscle contracture.

180

Palpation

- Warmth of a joint may be caused by inflammation, infection, or gout.
- Tenderness of a joint may be caused by injury, overuse, arthritis, inflammation, infection, or gout.

Mobile Joints—Range of Motion

- Limited range of motion in any joint may occur with bone or joint deformity or swelling, fracture, osteoarthritis, rheumatoid arthritis, idiopathic juvenile arthritis, or gout. Range of motion may also indicate voluntary (patient-controlled) restriction of movement due to pain or malingering.

Neurological

Proprioception/Cerebellar Function

- Inability to perform coordinated rapid alternating movements or other tests of coordination may be associated with muscle weakness, multiple sclerosis, conditions such as Parkinson's disease that cause tremors, or a cerebellar tumor.

Sensory Function

- Loss of accurate interpretation of sensation for stereognosis, graphesthesia, superficial touch, superficial pain, two-point discrimination, vibratory sensation, or position sense may indicate peripheral neuropathy or a brain disorder.

Superficial Reflexes

- A plantar or Babinski reflex is abnormal when the adult's great toe points upward and the other toes fan outward in response to the sole of the foot being stroked. An abnormal Babinski test may indicate a brain or a spinal cord lesion at level T7, T8, T9, T10, or T11.

Deep Tendon Reflexes (DTRs)

- A hypoactive or hyperactive DTR may suggest numerous disorders related to the associated spinal root, the central nervous system, an electrolyte imbalance, or a thyroid disorder.

Ankle Jerk Reflex

- Repetitive jerking of the calf muscle (clonus) may indicate meningitis, cerebral palsy, serotonin syndrome, or other disorder.

Index